DRUG REHABILITATION

How to Choose a Good Drug Rehab

Archie Nash

Websites:
drugrehabus.org
drugrehab.org.au

Published by: Archie Nash

Copyright Notice

Dedicated to my wonderful wife Margaret
whose support made this book possible.

TABLE OF CONTENTS

INTRODUCTION

This is not a book about drugs, or the inevitable consequences of drug use.

It is about taking a close hard look at the Drug Rehabilitation programs available to people who need them, and the importance of truly studying and assessing these programs.

It is hard to get a clear perspective when the different treatment options available have a purpose beyond just making the person drug free.

When they are influenced, or driven, by money, politics, self-interest, incomplete knowledge, even authority, what they offer can have very different outcomes.

So with all those factors at play, how do we make the call? What do we use to tell the difference between the good, the bad and the ugly? How do we pick a good drug rehab program?

The first thing we need to do is find out what rehabilitation really means.

The dictionary says:

Rehabilitate: to restore to a former capacity
: to restore to good repute
: to restore or bring to a condition
of health or useful and
constructive activity
Merriam-Webster Dictionary

Unless this happens at the end of a program one could say that the rehabilitation failed.

So how do we measure this?

Is there one common simple thing we can use to assess each and every rehab center?

Well, yes there is.

It is results.

After all, surely this is the only thing that matters anyway.

In the final analysis, results are the only true measure of success of any endeavor. Did you pass the exam? Did you win the match? Did you get the order?

Have you noticed that when you don't get a "yes" answer to that question you very quickly get given excuses or "reasons why" for the failure?

So the right question to keep in mind when doing research is: Are they getting results or are they giving me excuses?

Luckily, results can be measured. But when it comes to rehabs I have found it has to be measured in a certain way. Almost through the back door you might say.

Why?

Because I find that many rehabs disguise their true success rate.

Why on earth would they do that you may well ask?

Let me explain.

To see a rehab's true success rate it has to be done, not by just looking at their success rate, but by looking at the center's relapse rate as well.

That's right. Never just look at their "published success rate". While this can be helpful it is not enough on its own. You also have to look at their relapse rate. This is something not so well published, even hidden, fudged or given excuses for, by many centers that are not achieving rehabilitation by the above definition. The addict is NOT leaving the center, *returned to a former state of good health and constructive activity.*

So what is going on?

Say a person goes through a program and then falls over, in other words relapses, surely that is a program failure. I have found that reasons and excuses for these failures abound. But they are failures never-the-less and in many cases never counted.

Now relapse also needs to be defined. A Relapse is anybody who goes back to using drugs, or drinking alcohol to excess in the case of alcohol addiction, after doing a program. In other words, returning to usage or addiction again which means they were never really rehabilitated.

Whether they relapse minutes, days, weeks or months after the program is not the point. It is still a relapse and the program has failed.

By taking the time to conduct independent research on the success/relapse rate of many popular facilities, the common finding is not only discouraging, but scary. Almost any in-depth analysis will show that these programs have one thing in common, an incredibly high incidence of relapse. The figures are often not easy to see, but by doing a little bit of digging the all too common percentage for patients coming out of so many treatment models show a staggering 60% rate of relapse soon afterwards.

How do I get that figure? It's very simple. What they do, is count every person who leaves the program as a successful result. It works like this:
Many programs run for a set period of time. 30, 60, 90 days are common. When the time is up they send the person home. That is then counted as a result. If they relapse they sometimes come back and do the program again. When they are done that is another "result". The relapse part is not subtracted.

So what does this really mean? Well, for starters, it suggests that by merely completing the treatment, they claim a successful rehabilitation. This is an extreme example of course because they intentionally leave out the most important part:

Did the person stay off drugs or alcohol from then on? In other words were they, by definition, rehabilitated?

It is easy to place a person in a 30, 60, or even 90 day program – away from the possibility of using – and then once the predetermined timer runs out, releasing overly susceptible individuals back into a world full of temptation.

Now, temptation is a problem for so many people because it is something that requires a change within the individual to overcome. In fact, establishing a lasting breakthrough in the way the addict acts and thinks is the real challenge. Unfortunately, it is a challenge beyond the delivery capabilities of so many of the popular treatment methods.

As no institution likes to admit any holes in their program it is quickly dismissed as something that the addict must realize on his/her own. This type of funny logic, however, is very telling when you read between the lines. What is actually suggested by such a narrow-minded ideology is this: "Although we try to counsel, medicate, and encourage addicts to become drug-free, we really have no technique in place that is routinely successful in getting the person drug free, changing the way the addict thinks, lives, or changes him in a manner that is long lasting or permanent".

So, unfortunately what you are all-too-often left with is a brief period of abstinence while the addicted person is going through treatment; and upon release from treatment – with their body still containing residues of drugs and no new skills, attitudes or any life management strategies learned – your loved one is essentially a relapse waiting to happen. How can this possibly be called rehabilitation?

Drying out, getting clean, sobering up, or detoxification are all common ways of referring to the removal of toxic drugs from the body. However, the real situation is that metabolites* (little residues of the drug or drugs) can linger on in the body for great lengths of time, (up to years) despite cessation of drug taking.

The problem is that the idea of what constitutes actually becoming 'clean' is wildly misunderstood. To understand some of the principles covered I need you to get familiar with some terminology.

> **Metabolites**: comes from metabolism, which is: the process by which all living things turn food into energy and living tissue.
> **Metabolite**: a substance produced by metabolism.
> **World Book Dictionary**

You could say that metabolites are little bits or residuals left over from attempted metabolic digestion.

The difference between food and drugs

When a body is fed something it tests it to see what it is. If it can use it for nourishment then it treats it as food. If it is threatened by it, it tries to neutralize it or discharge it. Drugs are by definition poisons. This is a big surprise to many people. They never think of drugs this way.

> **Drug:** A substance (other than food) that, when taken into the body, produces a change in it. If the change helps the body the drug is a medicine, if the change harms the body, the drug is a poison.
> **World Book dictionary**

You can see from the definition, all drugs *change* the body and none of them are food. It is just that some don't do as much damage as others. Even medical drugs have what they call 'side effects' which is just another way of saying the effects we didn't want and we will have to put up with. What it comes down to is only a matter of quantity. A little bit of a drug like coffee or alcohol, aspirin, heroin, even morphine can give a person a boost, a lift, a kick. A bit more will put them to sleep. A lot more, all at the same time, will kill them. So a drug is basically and fundamentally a poison, clear and simple. Food does not do this no matter the quantity. Too much might make a person sick and throw up but that is a lot different from being poisoned.

Later on, we will take a look at the detoxification process more deeply and why it is crucial to success. The fact is there is more to a proper detox than simply not using for a while and waiting for the drugs to leave the body by themselves. In the chapters on detoxification I explain that there is much more to detoxification than simply 'waiting it out'.

Such 'waiting it out' while the body releases drug toxins is not enough. The explanation is not complicated, and is one of the biggest reasons that popular treatment options lose the battle, either in denial or being ignorant of the fact that metabolites of the toxins stay in the body longer than they are prepared to admit.

When a person returns to the outside world with such residuals still in the body, a release of these drug residuals are what causes a relapse the minute the person engages in any strenuous exercise or activity. Once this happens, the investment made into treatment is completely lost and your loved one is now back to square one: active addiction.

This phenomenon is now a well-established fact as a major cause of relapse, but is still refuted by the medical model. A true detox, as is fully explained later, will leave an addict completely free of these drug metabolites.

My goal in writing this book is to give a new sense of hope and a solution to desperate, worried family members and friends, whose lives have been seriously affected by the destructive nature of drug-abuse from those close to them. I have taken the time to investigate the most common treatment models, to dig into the literature and study case histories to find out why there is such an incredibly high rate of relapse and why the operators of some centers do not appear to make any effort to address the fundamental flaws in their program that bring about these failures.

By thoroughly examining all of the commonly used methods of drug treatment, I have found that there is one model in particular that not only achieves a higher success rate than all other models, but has a philosophy that, once investigated, proves to be not just a short-term deterrent to drug use, but rather a life-changing experience that works both in theory and in practice. In other words, a program that actually meets the full dictionary definition of rehabilitation.

This program is the Narconon program. It is unique, in that it does not have any of the self-imposed limitations to success that virtually all other models have. What I aim to do is present my research results that explain why the methods used in the Narconon model address and resolve the problems inherent in every other treatment program.

Through painstaking study, I have unearthed what a successful drug rehabilitation program must have and must deliver in order to truly achieve enduring success. The following, "Key Points" have been identified as the most important points to look for, and those to avoid if you want success in selecting a treatment center for your loved one. I can assure you that ignoring these findings will virtually guarantee a rehab failure.

1

TEN KEY POINTS THAT WILL REVEAL IF A REHAB WILL SUCCEED AND END ADDICTION

1. Participants need to stay as long as necessary.

Now, this may seem obvious, but too many treatments place a timer on the length of treatment. This is the first mistake. Addicts need to stay engaged in a program long enough to get the drugs fully out of their system and then after that they need to develop a life-changing mindset that will free them from repeating the mistakes they made in their past choices. They also need a routine to handle and remove the guilt and shame that comes to the surface as they come off the drugs. This needs to happen so that they can, with a clear conscience, face the people they hurt while addicted. In other words they have to get their self-respect back. Self-respect is the key personal attribute they lost at the time they began using. Unless they get their past poor choices cleaned up and become trustworthy again they will never be free as a person.

All this takes time. It is not possible to take a person who has been taking drugs sometimes for many years and, with the wave of a wand you might say, have them drug free in a few days. Just getting the drugs out of their system takes some time, never mind the time it takes to get them to address their past and look at where their decisions led them. Then they have to get some new understandings about themselves before there will be any change of attitude in the way they see things and their approach to daily life.

2. Withdrawal.

There is sometimes a lot of confusion between Withdrawal and detox

The withdrawal section is the first action that the person has to do. This is before anything else can possibly be considered. This is where the person actually comes off the drugs they are taking right now. It is not where the person becomes drug free or has the drugs taken out of their body. This is the first action before anything else can be done.

You cannot get the person's attention while they are totally under the influence of drugs. All you get is drug responses. This is not the same as detox. Detox is where the person has the drugs washed out of their system.

2

In the withdrawal section the person has to be very closely monitored. During this time the person will experience the full force and effect of the drugs and come up with every reason under the sun to run away and quit. This section takes considerable stamina from the addict and is almost impossible to do properly alone. As well as drugs, in the case of severe alcohol addiction, it is sometimes necessary to do a fully monitored medical withdrawal first before the person can be made stable and strong enough to be capable of doing a normal withdrawal. I only mention this point because alcohol is seldom considered to be a drug, let alone a drug that is all that serious. So it is a very good idea to discuss what the program offers in the way of withdrawal facilities and how they handle this critical aspect of the program. If the withdrawal phase is not done properly and effectively no further progress can be made.

Vital Requirement

There is vital requirement that must be done for the withdraw part of the program to work. Failing to do this will cause the addict far more pain than is necessary. Not only that, the withdrawal will fail and the addict will experience severe cravings and return to drug use shortly afterwards.

What happens is this: Drugs deplete the body of vital vitamins and minerals needed for it to function. If these aren't replaced, the person will experience severe craving. The main ones are calcium and magnesium. A person going through withdrawal must be given a measured amount of

3

these minerals and some vitamin supplements as well to get them safely off the drugs.

Not only that, there must be no drugs used during this withdrawal period as that will only keep the physical need going for more drugs.

So, the two key questions to ask any rehab center are, "Do you use drugs during the withdrawal stage, and what vitamins and minerals do you give to the addict as he goes through the withdrawal section". If they don't do this or refuse to answer the question, or worse, claim it is not necessary, then they don't know what they are doing, and the withdrawal they are offering is going to be very painful for your loved one and is not going to successfully get them off.

3. The Program MUST have an Effective Detox Phase.

This is critical otherwise a relapse is almost guaranteed.

One of the greatest problems with the majority of treatment facilities is that they do not provide a *proper* detoxification from drugs or alcohol. Most inpatient programs or attempts to dry out at home end up in relapse.

This is no longer a great mystery where we have to wonder why people get 'detoxed', only to return to drug use, weeks, months or years later.

4

The reason is actually very simple: only programs that provide an active detoxification will succeed in removing the actual *cause* of these seemingly endless relapses.

The reason for relapses are these drug metabolites which continue to linger in the individuals' fatty tissue, even long after the person has stopped using drugs.

The fact is, nearly all drugs are fat soluble. Certainly the most addictive are. This means that the drugs are attracted to the fatty tissues in the body and dissolve in them and stay there. It also means they can't be washed out with water as water and fat don't mix. Even when a heavy detox is done no matter how much water you drink the metabolites still remain in the fatty tissue.

In the case of a sauna detox, the bulk of the drugs will, without question, get released and the person will really feel that much better for it.

They might even feel they are now clean. However, that only half does the job as it still leaves these tiny residues in the fatty tissues ready to be released into the bloodstream the minute the person gets physically active and that is when the person again gets a taste of the drug and the craving starts all over again.

The residuals of the drugs linger, and eventually they *will* be released. This is a concept that only the Narconon program seems to actively address. It has and utilizes the only proven method of removing them, which is a program of replacement minerals and fats to wash out these tiny residues that are otherwise always left behind.

A typical, inpatient program does absolutely nothing to address this aspect of drug use, which has long been extensively studied and proven. So, without providing a means for the individual to rid these tiny toxins from their body, they are essentially leaving them apparently clean but really no more than a relapse waiting to happen.

Many other programs release their so-called 'patients' with the same amount of drug toxins in their body as they had on the day that they showed up. This is certainly the case with "replacement" drugs such as methadone. Replacing one drug for another is an admission of complete failure. It is definitely not making the person "drug free".

In the section entitled "Passive Detox vs. Active Detox" I provide an explanation to illustrate how imperative it is to use an active approach to drug detoxification. Without removing these residual toxins, the individual really isn't being fully 'detoxed'.

In contrast with the relapse-ridden histories of so many programs, it should be no surprise that your loved one may initially be skeptical of a different approach. However, the old cliché fits here. It is crazy to keep doing the same thing and expect a different result. The truth is: Only change changes things.

Yes, it is quite natural for your loved one to be wary of any detox since, in most cases, they are highly unpleasant and usually offer no real, long-term solutions. As a concerned parent, friend, or spouse, you can rest assured that the Narconon approach to detoxification is not only active and successful, but is a *true* detox in the sense that as well as removing the drugs from the person's body in general it also removes these leftover drug metabolites, something that is vital to achieve complete detox.

After students complete the Narconon detox, they are actually clean and free from drugs for the *very first time* since that first smoke of pot, or line of cocaine. Once they understand that it was these metabolites that were causing the earlier failures they will fully embrace the active detox method thus giving them the chance to become drug free and truly physically heal.

4. Replacing one addictive drug for another addictive drug is a recipe for failure.

Detox is a funny thing, because although most people *think* that they understand the process, there is more to it than most people think. The exact reasons why detox is the most important next step will be discussed in detail in the detox chapters.

The important thing to understand right now is that MORE drugs do not help anyone to detox. It acts completely in the OPPOSITE direction to the true goal of detox, which is: to remove all drugs and any lingering metabolites (bits of the

7

drug) from the body. These metabolites are a tricky thing to conquer, as they (literally) "stick" around much longer than most people realize.

The truth is they are stored in the fatty tissue of the body and later when the person engages in strong physical activities they get released back into the bloodstream, even after long periods of abstinence. In order to truly detox and give the person the best chance of a long sober or drug free life, the detox must be performed completely. This is a very precise routine and is based on a discovery that has been tested and proven to get consistent results for over 40 years of application in the field.

One can find arguments from supposed 'Authorities' decrying this discovery, claiming it is unscientific, claiming it is not proven, saying there is no "evidence" etc. However, the interesting thing is these same "authorities" and the programs based on their theories can't come within a mile of matching Narconon's results.

Surely "Authority" belongs only to those who can do the job. If you can't do the job you have no business calling yourself an authority.

Anyway, once a proper detox has been achieved, the only way a relapse is even possible is by re-introducing drugs into the now clean body. And as the saying goes – it would be all downhill again from there.

5. *Effective Life-Changing Attitudes, Personal Skills and Ability Development MUST be part of the Program.*

Without this section a return to old bad habits can easily happen.

Too many programs offer unsuccessful counseling and education that, while it may be informative, doesn't do anything to help the individual make better choices and ensure their sobriety is everlasting. Most treatment programs will discuss the effects of drugs and how they harm the body, etc. Well, this isn't really useful, as addicts *already* know this. It is redundant and a waste of very valuable time and resources.

Additionally, programs need to give their participants a way to overcome the guilt and shame they carry because of what they did while using. Students of Narconon are given a way to own up to their mistakes of the past.

This action allows them to move on from past feelings of guilt or shame.

If such issues are not addressed, then it leaves the door open to the possibility of the person going back to their old ways despite the fact that they are now physically clean.

The program must have a section that relieves the addict from feeling ashamed of the things that he/she has done. Certainly, there is no reward for the bad things that they have done during their addiction, but it must be something that they acknowledge, understand, and take

9

responsibility for so they can move on from their past.

By taking stock of the events that happened to them, only then are they able to move on to a life that is not only sober, but also emotionally clean as well and free from guilt.

6. Located away from Urban Areas is better.

It is a sad and unfortunate fact that many inpatient facilities have what might be best described as "run-aways" who leave the center and disappear as soon as they can. Even when they have entered with high hopes and determination to do a program, in the beginning the drugs are still in control.

This can make them want to run-away even as they detox, especially when the drug influence becomes even stronger as the drugs start to come out of their system.

Running away is less likely to happen if the center is well removed from a major metropolitan area where escaping into the wilderness is far less attractive. Not only that, in a large city, there are inevitably drugs, and believe it or not, many users are quite comfortable to search out the worst neighborhoods even in an unfamiliar city to score drugs. It happens all the time and this brings on some of the worst activities imaginable, because without money, the addict will often resort to crime

10

such as theft or prostitution in order to get money in an unfamiliar area. Arrests are common. Overdoses, weeks or months without contact or hearing from them are all too common. This can be an extremely sad ordeal.

That is why, in order to remove the temptation of easily getting drugs that might be only walking distance away, the center should not be in an urban environment. Addicts will happily buy drugs from strangers, and this invites other undesirable outcomes.

The fact remains that every large city in the United States has a drug problem. It is not a good idea to provide someone with rehabilitation in the same place where they can easily get drugs and where simply giving up seems like a reasonable option.

While not critical, it is far, far better to remove that option and select a center that is away from a city. Even better is to go to a rehab in another state where the patient has no known drug dealers or contacts at all.

7. Programs Should Offer External Support.

The student must be able to receive support, encouragement, and have contacts in place to serve any emotional need.

Support must be everlasting just as sobriety itself must be. Family visits can help a lot, and oddly, many inpatient facilities do not allow this for reasons that make no real sense. Family support is crucial, and the successful center will encourage support not only from the inside through staff, but also from outside in the form of visits by friends, family, and significant others.

Narconon encourages all graduates to reach out to the center anytime they feel the need. This is often a rewarding moment for staff members as well as students. Many times, even years after treatment, the phone will ring and a former student will be on the line.

Most times these students may wish to talk to a favorite staff member and simply thank them for the power that has been given back to them, along with the life-changing realizations that they have made and applied to their life post-treatment. In such events Narconon staffs are eager to hear about how former students have been getting along, and can offer suggestions for maintaining the great life they have been living since their graduation from the program.

If a center doesn't have an open welcome line for their students after treatment, it sends a message to the person that they never really cared about their sobriety to begin with. An open line to the center is essential for former students: whether to help them through a rough patch in their lives, or conversely to congratulate them on their success and offer suggestions on how to keep up the great work. Having this shows students that they are important to the program, not only when they are actively enrolled, but from there on out.

8. A Treatment Program should be Open to People of Any and Every Culture, Race, Religion.
Non-Secular Programs Can Be Restrictive

This may seem obvious to some readers, and it *should* be obvious. However, many programs that do not offer a secular approach not only limit their own reach in who they allow to participate, but also may not appeal to the person who is considering attending.

The center needs to be open and welcoming to ALL people and not limit itself to one particular demographic. Addiction is a condition that affects people of all cultures, religions, and races. It is no more than a condition, which unlike a disease, does not spread nor is it contagious.

However, it is often helpful for people of different and diverse backgrounds to come together to overcome a common problem.

That is one of the great things about the Narconon program. It allows people of different backgrounds to come together, learn together, and heal together. It promotes a healthy bond between people who may appear to be different or have different beliefs, but find out they have much more in common than they may have originally thought. This is not only beneficial while going through the program, but also promotes a sense of unity among people that goes far beyond their time in treatment.

Students of Narconon make new friends, learn from each other, and develop a stronger bond between students than any other program ever could.

This is a common problem for people who would like to attend A.A. or N.A. meetings: they are worried about not fitting in with the group, and if they feel they are going to be judged or treated differently from the start, then they have already lost hope in the program before even engaging in it. Successful programs will not only welcome people of all backgrounds, but also actively encourage a diverse population. This allows your loved one to not have to worry about who they are, where they come from, or what they look like on the surface. They need to be encouraged that the common denominator that brought them to treatment is an addiction that can, and will, be overcome.

This itself brings a sense of unity to their treatment, so they can be comfortable in working with one another, despite any small, insignificant differences, and work together and learn together to overcome the *one* thing that they all have in common: a dependency on drugs or alcohol.

Not only is a non-secular approach important during treatment itself, but also as many new friends are made through successful treatments, students will have a wide-range of new friends whom they can rely on when they become drug free.

Many friendships are made during treatment programs and Narconon graduates are quite often keen to stay in touch with each other post treatment.

14

This is encouraging to the student, as they realize that despite all the bad things they may have done, they still have a supportive outside network of friends who care about them and are hoping for better times for them.

Basically, the non-secular approach is farther-reaching than just during treatment. It is often the start of many lifelong friendships that are formed with a common new outlook on life, encouraging unification and progress among students, rather than being divisive.

There is another interesting aspect to this which is not culture related but is quite a factor. When the person becomes drug free they do need new drug free friends. When they finish the program they have no desire to go back to their old drug "friends" unless it is to try to rescue them the way they have been rescued. Bonding with other graduates is the start of a new circle of drug free friends with very solid and common values and is quite therapeutic in itself.

9. The Program Should Not Require Repeat Enrollment to Work.

If it has done its job properly, that should be the end of it.

Far too many programs leave addicts behind the moment they walk out the door, even if the staff suspects that the person will struggle – many simply do not offer aftercare. For the ones that do, the best they can usually offer is just more of the same -- which by the very fact that they are back means that the program never delivered.

The Narconon program doesn't have as a requirement that students return to the program. Once it is completed the graduates are ready to enter the world again, with confidence. Still, support is available should a graduate have a problem. While this is rare for graduates, it *is* available to them.

Even things as simple as talking to a favorite staff member on the phone can do wonders for a person's confidence and assurance that the program actually and truly cares about them and their sobriety.

They are not just a number, a patient, or thought of as no more than profit to the organization. They are a student who has learned much, but if they have a problem they need to know that they can always reach out knowing someone on staff will always be able to come up with a good solution.

When Narconon graduates leave the program it is rare that they ever need to come back to the program. This is what becoming a graduate really means. It means the person has graduated from being a drug addict to being a drug free decent human being again and able to live his life under his own determination as a productive and useful person. In other words he is truly rehabilitated.

10. A Program Should Deliver a Drug Free Person Fully Rehabilitated and Equipped with life skills to Succeed.

No matter how long an addict needs to complete the program – timeframes are not a measure of success. 30 days, 28 days, 60 days, 90 days, 6 days, or 3 months – do you see a pattern here? What do these numbers all have in common? Well, I suppose that is a trick question, as the answer is that they have absolutely nothing in common. If you explain the situation which you are in with your addicted loved one, to 10 different 'experts' you can expect at least 8 different recommendations for the best program.

Now, the normal opinion between experts on an objective subject is to come up with the same conclusions regarding effective treatment. Two physicians shown medical disease symptoms such as, say, measles will pretty much come up with the same diagnosis and treatment– it is objective and the science of medical disease diagnosis is common, well understood and universal.

Pose a similar problem to two 'experts' in support of a disease based addiction model, and you will get wildly different suggestions, diagnoses, and prognoses – followed by wildly different treatment recommendations and the time needed for treatment. Why is the field of addiction treatment so unpredictable and so different from normal diseases?

When closely inspecting the 'disease' theory model, you quickly discover the shameless

17

similarities to the corporate business model. The main goal for a business is profit generation. The hard, unfortunate truth is that the 'disease' model of treatment actually benefits from failed sobriety and relapses because this becomes repeat business.

A treatment program that offers a fixed, single payment says a lot about the sincerity of the center. If a center really wanted to recover and more often than not save the life of your friend or family member who has gone off the rails into addiction, they would be more interested in the result than in the money.

A fixed price, without any limitation on the length of stay shows enquiring families that although money is necessary to pay running costs, that is the only factor in their fee structure and there is no other financial motivation. Such programs have a unique sincerity and empathy for helping people overcome their addictions. A program that follows such a regime considers 'repeat business' to be a program failure, not a financial opportunity.

When deciding on a treatment facility, consider this: will they take your hard-earned money, and then 30 days later release a walking, talking relapse waiting to happen? Or will they work with the individual until they are confident that the person is drug free not only for the moment, but also that the person will stay drug free 5, 10, or more years later.

Most programs avoid presenting their statistics or any numbers at all, about the relapse rate of their patients. This is certainly mysterious, but when considered from a business point of view it suddenly makes sense for a dollar-driven program. The long-term success rate, held by the Narconon organization, is in the range of over 70%.

This is incredibly impressive, as this figure is actually higher than the high-school graduate rate in many areas in the U.S. The embarrassingly low numbers of practically every other treatment model suggest that they simply do not work.

The truth is, a model is not 'working' if it does not routinely achieve a high rate of success, with only a few, isolated cases of relapse. A stunning statistic is that the relapse rate for the Narconon program is actually roughly the same as the average true success rate for most other programs. To reiterate this extremely important fact, and to put it the other way around – the success of Narconon, even at the low end of 70%, is almost the same as the FAILURE rate of most other programs.

This can be attributed to four main factors:
a) The others don't actually HAVE a full understanding of how to get a person drug free.
b) They don't know how to do a complete detox to prevent relapse.
c) They offer no relief to free the person from their past life style and transgressions against their friends and others.
d) They don't have or include any workable life skills to enable the addict to change his attitude and be able to lead an honest and successful drug free life.

Given the need for a life changing personal transformation to counteract the likelihood of relapse as being just about the most important ability that an addict needs to acquire and master, it begs the question as to why all programs don't focus on this aspect and have in place proven activities to achieve this skill.

Could it be they don't know how? In looking into any rehab program it should act as a huge warning sign if they are unable or unwilling to provide any data of long-term success rates. If they can't, it can be taken to mean one of two things:

1) The data does exist, but is too embarrassingly low and thus needs to be kept hidden, or

2) They don't track and keep the data, which is equally concerning, because this is the only true measure of success.

2

Programs in General

Despite many options, inpatient treatment is the most chosen and popular model by not only families, but also the judicial system. While this in itself is a good idea and the intentions, on behalf of families and judges, are actually sincere, their lack of knowledge or wrong knowledge on the subject of detox, rehabilitation and what really works can lead them to choose ineffective programs when making a decision on the best place to send their loved one or to send an offender.

Inpatient facilities often publish and can appear to have the right intentions, but many models are simply completely off-base and flawed. Typically they follow the so-called "medical model", basing their own program on academia's disease model. This is a huge mistake. Apart from the fact that drug addiction is not a disease, academia base their assumptions on what they believe or hope will work **in theory**, not what actually works **in practice**. These two words are extremely important considerations when deciding on a treatment program. Inpatient models everywhere have absolutely embarrassing relapse rates – so far from acceptable, that most programs go out of their way to hide their statistics regarding relapse.

By doing a bit of independent research, you will find that often the 'best' success rates (meaning, no post-treatment relapses) come in at around 25%, and the worst at a staggering 10% success rate. What are these treatment programs doing with your money and invested time and hope? According to the numbers, not very much, because this is an appalling statistic.

In the United States, prisons are grossly overcrowded. In an attempt to cut back on expenditure in the criminal justice system – in which a single inmate costs approximately $30,000 per year – many judicial systems decide, overzealously, that an inpatient treatment center is a good option. This removes the offending addict from the streets for a short period of time; it certainly saves jail space, while at the same time they believe they are giving the offender a chance at rehabilitation. This is fundamentally a good idea and would be very effective if the rehab center they were sent to did its job and got the offender drug free.

There are two aspects to this deal.

One is the centers they get sent to are usually the medical/establishment model with its appalling relapse rate and the other is you cannot rehab the unwilling.

This is a sad state of affairs because, in the main, judges are restricted to sending offenders only to medical model type centers so the offender is soon back on the streets unchanged and the other is that no one can help or change a person who is unwilling to take part, not even Narconon.

Quite often the offender is no more ready for rehab than a fly is ready to die when you swat at it. I probably need to make this point again because it is a key factor in any person's attitude. It seems no one can make an unwilling person do something they absolutely refuse to do. If you do not have their co-operation nothing will be achieved and no progress can be made. A person can be made to go through the motions of doing something, but unless they are contributing to the motion and at least trying nothing will happen.

The addict, of course, will always resist facing up to their situation as that is part of what drugs do to the person. The skill of the intake councilor is in getting the person to face up to their situation and bring about in them a willingness to enter rehab and give it their best shot. Make no mistake this is a high level skill. Parents and friends are usually too close to the addict to bring this about, such is their emotional involvement. They certainly *can* do it, but it is not common.

I just need to point out that you may be tempted to follow the example of locally appointed and respected judges and assume that if this is what they are doing it must be the right action to follow for the regular family with an addicted person problem.

The judicial system is one thing but the addicted person whom you love deserves more

23

attention and care than the revolving door that is the Western criminal justice system. There is no effective drug rehab in any jail.

Outside of jail, and taking into account the high relapse rates of most inpatient facilities, it eventually becomes clear that there is something extremely wrong with their model of treatment. "But where are the GOOD treatment programs?" you may well ask. "Why haven't I heard about the programs that actually work long-term?"

Now we come to the factor of the establishment. Pushing the disease model as they do allows them to push even more drugs. There is a huge vested interest in the medical model.

They are promoted, pushed, funded and supported by interests that get huge government allocations and commercial profits to keep them going. Success is not the main purpose of their operation even though they adamantly assert that it is.

Drug manufacturing companies stand to get a never ending stream of orders for methadone or any other drug they can develop and claim "neutralizes" addiction drugs. In cahoots with psychiatrists they can go on forever claiming they are nearly there with a solution if they just had a bit more time and money to keep researching and trialing.

The fact is they have been making this claim since drug addiction began and all they have to show for it are the appalling relapse rates listed above. The last thing they want is a truly successful program. They will scream and yell and deny and try to discredit any evidence that shows up their money making scheme. If they really wanted to handle the drug problem they would be delighted to find and welcome anyone or anything that could show a better rate of success and a lower rate of relapse.

Instead Narconon suffers considerable attack from this source. Considering the exemplary and proven success rate of Narconon for over 45 years it begs the question as to what are the motives and intentions of those behind the big pharma/psychiatrist/pseudo medical model. Actually, you could say, it confirms the proposition that the last thing they want is a workable effective solution.

In addition, non-medical model programs with extremely low rates of relapse, such as Narconon, rarely have a coalition of eager ex-addicts willing to do public or media interviews. Mostly this is because ex-addicts don't want to suffer this same kind of cruel and vicious attack. Yes, they certainly tell their friends, but high profile announcements, media exposure and the publicity from story seeking journalists is not generally a part of what they want to get into in their new life.

This is extremely unfortunate for the majority, who need to know about such available options, but from the standpoint of a former addict who has completed the program and lives a happy, healthy life, the last thing he wants is to revisit the low points of his life. It's not about shame either, but there is an underlying tendency for happy people to be happy in silence about their past.

Uncovering this 'happy silence' is one of the motivations for writing this book. Too many people are not even aware that great programs are even out there. Additionally, due to programs like Narconon being sincere, and not interested in getting into smear campaigns themselves, they just get on with doing their job and let the vested interests waste their millions on black PR campaigns.

It is a very interesting truism of life that an accuser will always accuse the other person of what he is up to himself in an attempt to shift attention off his hidden deeds so (he thinks) he won't be discovered. Husbands and wives can be seen playing this game when there has been cheating going on. One accusing the other of what they have been doing themselves.

3

The Legal Fix That Doesn't Fix – Maintenance Therapy

Unfortunately, replacement therapy for opiate/opioid dependency is becoming an increasingly popular strategy. From an addicts' perspective to be allowed to keep chemicals in his system 24/7 without any legal repercussions and even with medical encouragement can seem like a great idea. Although an honest physician would have to agree that even from a medical perspective, this is nothing more than a drug-for-drug tradeoff. Methadone and Buprenorphine (Suboxone, Subutex) are some of the strongest narcotics available to an addict. Not only are they constantly abused, but such abuse is easily hidden while the treatment façade protects the addict from owning up to any of his or her problems.

The extremely sad truth is that doctors become the equivalent of drug dealers when these methods are used. It is not treatment, by any honest standard of the word. The real issues are completely abandoned when a person chooses to participate in such programs, and the problem of dependency is prolonged and more often than not becomes much worse. So why are these methods gaining more participation? There are several reasons:

Availability – A person's environment is often an enormous trigger for continued drug use. For instance, what does a nearby clinic or doctor, which the addict knows will provide him with a legal, sustainable drug, really become? That's right, just another supplier. The addict and even an uninformed family can trick themselves into thinking that this backwards approach is a sensible option. The fact is these methadone and Suboxone doctors are essentially nothing more than another variety of drug dealer. In fact, in the case of public programs, they are drug dealers who are being paid with public tax dollars. These private clinics and public pharmacies sell their wares in a building rather than on the street-corner. So, really you have two situations: public tax dollars providing drugs, or private enterprise profiting by sustaining addictions.

Fear - Addicts know that narcotic withdrawal reactions are non-life threatening even at their worst, but they suffer a sense of fear from the idea of going through a withdrawal followed by complete abstinence. It is a truly selfish perspective to continue using another drug, based on a cowardly fear of going through physical withdrawal and the reactions that brings on. Such reactions are unpleasant, yes, but are to be an expected result while coming off the chemicals that have been accruing and building up to unmanageable addiction. By remaining stoned, the damaged brain does not heal, nor does the person. Rather, a dulled state of mental catatonia is maintained under the guise of treatment.

Misinformation – Perhaps the biggest contributor to this awful trend is misinformation. Addicts may see another fellow addict start methadone and no longer hang out at in the streets. This may give the extremely false perception that the person has improved his life somehow. This fallacy is the biggest problem because being misinformed it tricks the person into believing that he will make progress. If a loved one of yours is considering maintenance therapy, ask him what will happen next in his progression to a healthy life. They will not have an answer, because there is no progression or next step up. They are showing you that they can't think ahead and have not thought it all the way though at all. This is standard brain- affected drug talk. They are only thinking of a different habit that is not so much taboo.

No Real Goals – This one is hard for some to swallow, but the fact is that there is no benefit in replacing one drug for a different drug. No recovered ability or goal setting can ever come out of doing that. A chemical filled brain does not think clearly or logically. A person can't set future goals in this condition. The effects of the earlier drugs are still there if no detox is done and now you have this new replacement drug adding to the damage done by the earlier drug. It just becomes an accumulation of more drug toxins, so the truth is that these substitute or replacement programs actually make the transition to a sober life *much* more difficult. It is just continued toxification to the addict.

This crazy routine actually extends the length of dependency. This is not treatment or rehabilitation of any sort. It is no more than a trumped-up legal fix for the addict under the false assumption that because a nurse or pharmacist dispenses the drugs they are suddenly of some use or an appropriate medicine.

You don't treat addiction with medicine or drugs of any sort because that is only going to be counter-productive, costly, and continue the addiction. In fact it only makes matters worse because it adds to the chance of becoming even more addicted and certainly causes more residual build-up.

Since addiction is not a disease in the true sense of the word 'disease', medicine is not going to make any difference to the condition but will only make it worse. It's the wrong solution for the problem so can never work. These replacement drugs are only variations if not just the same as the drugs that are used on the street anyway and many addicts simply go straight out and sell their so-called 'treatment' on the street.

Consider this, how many people are selling their insulin on the street to diabetes patients who actually have the disease? None of course. Just the fact that these medications end up on the black market itself should be a big clue that they are not helpful to the addict or anybody else except maybe the companies that profit from pushing them.

The Wrong Environment – Countless undercover sting operations have occurred not only on the seedy streets of major U.S. cities, but also at methadone and Suboxone clinics. Undercover surveillance and investigative news outlets have also documented what often becomes an open-air drug market. "Well, that makes no sense...", you may be thinking, but it's very much a reality. In some areas with especially high heroin problems, such as Baltimore, Maryland (perhaps the heroin capital of the United States – ironically less than an hours drive from the Nation's Capital) where the population of drug users is staggering, these 'clinics' have become a trading post for all sorts of drugs. Methadone is often sold in exchange for heroin, crack, or PCP not even out of sight of these actual clinics. In fact, many dealers in Baltimore will hang out near methadone clinics, and who can blame them? Some of their best customers are going in and out the doors every day.

At a clinic near Philadelphia, an undercover news operation actually caught the following on video: a female enters the methadone clinic. Outside the clinic many people are hanging around, and many of them don't ever go inside. Shortly thereafter, the female returns outside after receiving her daily dose of the legal narcotic methadone.

She is then observed accepting money from another individual just 'hanging out' near the clinic. After receiving the money, the female who entered the clinic spits in a Styrofoam cup and hands it to the person who provided the money who quickly drinks it up.

31

What just happened in this situation? Well, since so many methadone 'patients' consistently fail drug tests, some clinics force them to take the methadone under supervision (except on the weekends – everyone takes the drug home on Saturday, no matter how many failed urine tests).

So this female pretending to drink the methadone provided by the clinic held it in her mouth, walked outside, and sold it to another person who drank the methadone instead – directly from the addict's mouth. The spit I'm assuming was no charge. This is not only illegal, fraudulent, and an exploitation of a terrible form of 'treatment', but also dangerous.

What happens if the person who buys the methadone cannot tolerate an especially high dose? They may drop dead. What happens to the female who sold her legal fix along with her spit? She probably went around the corner to a street-dealer awaiting someone just like her, and purchased some heroin with the money that she gained by selling her so-called 'medicine'.

No other real disease has any medicine that people would sell on the streets. I can't recall ever hearing of a person selling antibiotics on a street corner, or insulin – although the insulin syringes make it to the street, unfortunately. The reason why insulin and antibiotics are not sold openly on the street in major cities across the country is because there is no underground market for actual medicine. None.

So, what are these clinics providing for their 'patients' that makes the 'medicine' have such a high value on a street corner? That's a trick question really, because these drugs are not medicine, they are drugs of abuse and drugs of addiction. Real medicine is not hocked in alleys, it is provided by a pharmacist in a shop.

There is an exception though, and that is another narcotic that comes from the pharmacies as well. This is Suboxone, a newer narcotic drug similar to methadone.

The funny thing about Suboxone is that it is usually an expensive medication to acquire. A single pill may sell for about $10 at a pharmacy. On the streets of Baltimore, where out of 600,000 residents about 60,000 are drug addicts – yes, that's 1 out of every 10 people – you will find these Suboxone pills sell on the street for $5. Now, that doesn't seem to make sense does it? Why would a greedy drug dealer sell a drug for less than he may have paid for it? Yes, another trick question – he didn't pay for it, tax dollars paid for his prescription. Taxes paid for the narcotic that is so over-prescribed that it allows dealers to actually charge less than the pharmacy does.

I am honestly convinced that substituting one drug for another is probably the absolute **worst** option to choose. Don't feel bad if you have fallen into this trap with a loved one yourself however, because there is so much misinformation around that actually gives these certified drug-dealers credit. The reality is that these maintenance drugs should be renounced as much as the illicit drugs are themselves – the end results are the same, and don't be fooled by doctor's 'opinions' on this subject either.

Replacing one drug for another drug continues the cycle of addiction and doesn't address the real problem that is causing the habit, so the person can never break the habit and therefore will never get to live drug free.

Think about what some doctors rely on for their livelihoods. Could it be a steady supply of revenue from addicted patients who absolutely need to see them and spend lots of money in order to do what? Well, stay an addict of course.

Yes, that's exactly what happens, and the patient taking Suboxone or Methadone – which are becoming dangerously popular treatment choices (and now are street drugs as well) – are quite possibly the best long term customers for a doctor, pharmacist, or clinic. The only thing that is different is the location and the clothes that these 'professionals' wear – their role is exactly the same as the shady guy on the street corner pushing hard drugs. This should be considered a scam and a scandal by anyone who wants *real* sobriety for their loved one. It's just another drug outlet trying to disguise itself as something that it isn't: legitimate treatment/rehabilitation.

Maintenance is an admission of total failure to achieve any kind of rehabilitation whatsoever.

How can a person be 'rehabilitated' if they are still taking drugs, no matter what the drug is?

4

The Fallacy of the Disease Model

We have already discovered that the relapse rate from the medical model is extremely high so this fact alone shows it is a failed program. That should be enough really just by itself.

But consider this: If it was a disease then it would respond to medication like any other disease. However, in practice, using the disease model idea all we get is relapse after relapse after relapse.

They explain these relapses away by saying the "medication" failed or it was wrong or it is a genetic fault or comes from some kind of neurochemical imbalance and that there is no real cure. If the addict suicides they claim they didn't get to them soon enough. How soon is soon enough?

Well to anyone who has not taken the trouble to study their performance results, this might seem a reasonable explanation. But this excuse has been going on for years and years and years. Surely after all this time of testing and research they would have found something that worked. But no, their results in getting people off drugs are no better today than they were 50 years ago.

Clinging to the "addiction is a disease" concept is an incredibly narrow view and leaves them with no other choice than the use of drugs to handle the problem. This begs the question of why won't they consider any other proposition.

They never seem to question their fundamental assumption as a reason for why they fail all the time. This is another red alert. If someone was genuine they would look at and question every aspect of their activity all the way down to their basic assumptions.

The outcomes of this disease philosophy i.e. relapse after relapse after relapse are so easy to observe that I encourage anyone interested enough to make the observation as I did. It is also quite easy to observe a person who has become drug free, is staying drug free and is living a revitalized new life. If these former addicts now drug free, truly had a disease of any sort to begin with, one would expect to see the medical establishment demanding to know what they had done to get "cured" and what the medicine or program was that had 'cured' them. This is if they were truly interested in ending drug addiction.

However, the medical model group asserts that such a successful and happy person isn't really cured at all and is still inflicted with the 'disease' and will be for the rest of their life and any abstinence is, at best, only temporary. Of course they would say this because that is all that happens in their program.

It would be a laughable concept if the stakes weren't so high, but given the seriousness of the matter this potential comedy is nothing short of a tragedy. For right there, those people who have faith in medicine as a cure-all are immediately compromised by calling addiction a disease.

It is a terrifying idea when you really think about it: A disease for which there is not only no cure, but also no objective way to measure it or treat it. If it can't be measured or seen under a microscope how do they know it is a disease?

If drug addiction was an actual disease it would show up in an x-ray or under a microscope or some other standard common medical test.

If it has no cure how then do they explain the thousands of examples of former drug users who have been successfully rehabilitated by a different non-medical model program and who have never returned to drug use?

Even worse, this grossly incorrect term 'disease model' is in conflict with the actual definition of what constitutes a disease!

Disease, "dis-ease, **n**. a disorder of structure or function in a human, animal, or plant, esp. one that produces specific signs or symptoms or that affects a specific location and is not simply a direct result of physical injury: *bacterial meningitis is a rare disease / a possible cause of heart disease.*"

That is the actual terminology that SHOULD be used when speaking of any disease. Drug addiction clearly does not fit within those parameters. So, how do they get away with the usage applied to addiction? Easy, unfortunately, as the same dictionary also recognizes and explains figurative language use as well, and after giving the proper, medical definition, the New Oxford American Dictionary highlights the following, in bold no less (perhaps because it is an important consideration that is often overlooked), directly beneath the previous, proper terminology

"<Special Usage> *FIGURATIVE* a particular quality, habit, or disposition regarded as adversely affecting a person or group of people: *departmental administration has often led to the dread disease of departmentalitis.*"

It is clear that there are two ways to use the word – however, when speaking in a medical or academic manner, it is simply unprofessional to knowingly combine the very different literal and figurative definitions of what a 'disease' really is. It appears that the literal term obviously does not fit as a definition for drug addiction.

By using a figurative manner of speech to call addiction a 'disease', not only is the word

38

disease being bent and molded to shape the needs of the medical model proponents who have no clue about how to cure it but the extremely important difference between literal meaning and figurative meaning gets blurred in the public mind.

Any program that uses a 'disease' model for addiction will readily admit defeat (though not in such everyday terms, of course) by saying there is no cure.

This is entirely FALSE! There is a cure, but it is simply not seen by the eyes of the kind of doctors and academics who are riding on the disease model bandwagon. With eyes wide shut, and strutting their authority they claim addiction is a disease and that there is no cure.

To a desperate mother, family or spouse, what sort of a heartbreak announcement is that?

Hopefully, by understanding the nature of what the 'disease' model truly implies you won't go down that road, or get lured into that trap.

The thing is, there *is* a way to end addiction – and it is becoming more and more widely recognized for the diamond it really is. In the next few years, as drug use continues to soar, you will find that Narconon will become the Rehabilitation Program of choice by those who really care.

Unfortunately, I also know that until more family members and loved ones discover and experience the transformation of their formerly addicted friend, spouse, or child made drug free

39

and rehabilitated, by dictionary definition, Narconon will still appear to be the secret success that despite its open doors, people will have to look for to find.

Narconon reaches out as much as it can, but it is usually only after families have endured the mental frustration of continued failures elsewhere that they finally come to the organization, often in utter desperation. This is sad because they could have saved themselves a lot of wasted time and money, never mind the unnecessary suffering, which their loved one has had to endure by not coming sooner.

5

A.A. / N.A. Meetings: Taking a Leap of Faith
Why it's not worth the risk

Anyone familiar with the meetings of Alcoholics Anonymous or Narcotics Anonymous (A.A. and N.A. respectively) can probably understand the first line of the title of this section and its relevance. You may not understand the potential risks, however. There are many reasons why these programs are so popular, and some of them are noble in their own regard or intentions – there is no monetary motivation, and the ideology seems sincere enough – so what could be such a risky leap of faith.

Perhaps more accurately, it's more than a little leap, such as jumping over a small puddle. Rather, more like an Olympics record length long jump. There are so many potential errors in this type of treatment, if you even call it a 'treatment' at all. More accurately, these programs are just a social networking support system that attempts to bring alcoholics and addicts together to encourage one another to remain sober. The basis of each program is the same and involves following a 12 step model, in which participants are encouraged to complete each step in succession.

This model of program is, for some, a turnoff right from the start, as there is a strong religious element to it. Now, I'm not suggesting that faith is not an important thing. In fact if the addict hasn't at least got faith in himself he will never make it through any program. But for many this religious aspect is unappealing. The overly strong surrender to a 'higher power' that is required by the program has lost the interest of many young and sometimes religiously uncertain people right from the very start.

That is not the major problem though with these meetings. The meetings, unfortunately, have no internal structure –aside from the 12 steps. Any sort of formal structure or plan is completely absent. In addition, there are no trained professionals present to help guide your loved ones in the right direction. There is nothing to address the necessity of proper detoxification, which alone makes it not even a feasible proposition. Until they have already achieved a proper active detoxification – which, really is only obtained through the Narconon treatment model – attending these meetings will do nothing to prevent relapse.

The problem is the lack of order, structure, or guidance and any game plan aside from the 12 steps. This means that when a participant brings up a problem there is no standard routine to handle it or help them. There is no consistency to the program aside from the prayers. Whilst participation in prayers is encouraged they yet remain voluntary.

Although the meetings *do* get one thing right, which is a strict adherence to sobriety, they don't actually follow through or enforce it in any way, shape, or form – and are powerless to do so, by and large. Vocalizing criticism is about as far as it goes, and the person is still encouraged to return to the next meeting.

It is also an unwelcome fact that some people actually do attend these meetings while drunk or under the influence of drugs (I have witnessed it myself, sadly), and when it is noticed it is surely frowned upon, but that's really about it. There is just no structure to prevent this sort of behavior at a meeting.

There is also this terrible little secret, which many adherents would rather blindly ignore than address and it is this: some people, especially upon meeting new people in a non-controlled environment, actually use the setting as a meet-and-greet for new drug connections and finding new dealers and even new drugs. Think about it for a moment. What a wonderful opportunity to find new contacts when you are surrounded by people in the same condition as yourself.

While the following may be a hypothetical example of this activity, from what I have seen I believe it goes something like this:

A young person, let's call him Jason, may very well walk in to a N.A. meeting having recently completed a (passive) detox at home. Soon, as he's listening to the group of participants in the large circle of chairs facing each other relate their stories, he notices an attractive girl who is 'nodding off' slightly. To the untrained eye, this may seem like someone who hasn't had enough sleep.

Nothing to worry about, maybe she didn't get much sleep the night before, or just doesn't drink the gallons of coffee typically consumed at such meetings. Jason is truly committed to staying clean, that's why he decides to try the N.A. meetings in the first place. Throughout the meeting stories are shared, in great and specific detail, about the trouble that drugs have caused them throughout their lives. Some are tragic, some may be funny (to the group, I wouldn't imply any story about addiction is 'funny'), some may even (intentionally or not) glorify past drug use. Jason is new and shy around the group of strangers, so he doesn't participate in the war stories – and this is OK, the group accepts that from new members and is simply happy he is there – but he does notice the unfamiliar, yet attractive girl again scratching her nose and face.

Eventually, upon her turn to speak, the attractive girl introduces herself as an addict. She is greeted with a cheerful chorus throughout the group, "Hello Jennifer!" Then, Jennifer goes on to tell everyone that she is celebrating her first 90 days clean TODAY! Everyone claps and one member gives her a special bracelet to wear, to show her sober pride. She is happy, and quickly takes her seat again, still scratching her face ever so subtlety from time to time, and dozing off here and there.

The stories continue around the circle, and Jason isn't paying attention much to what anyone is saying. He is fixated on Jennifer, and it is not an interest in any human flesh that is invading his mind. He is watching closely, not sure if he is the only one who sees her subtle behavior. His brain automatically radars in on it, being only 'clean' for a few weeks, the metabolites of the heroin still hiding in his fat cells begin to make his muscles tense, and his palms are clammy. He doesn't know it, but his pupils begin to dilate to twice their size – an ocean of black with a slight ring of blue around it. The meeting adjourns after the ending prayer, but Jason left a minute before, excusing himself to the restroom. He enters and his stomach is churning. He feels sick; he feels 'dope-sick', as he had for a week while he kicked the heroin at home cold turkey only 2 months ago. He splashes his face with water, notices his pupil size in amazement, and then hurries outside to light up a smoke.

He swivels his head through the crowd that has exited and sees Jennifer walking in the exact opposite direction from his destination. Quickly, he runs to catch up to her, as she is descending down the subway stairs, "Hey there!" he exclaims with enthusiasm. She turns her head and offers a cheery, but awkward, "Oh, hello, you're the new guy that was at..." before she even finishes the sentence Jason interrupts her, "So congratulations on your 90 days clean, you look like you're doing good, want to celebrate? My treat." Jennifer immediately recognizes the unspoken sarcasm to his words "you look good", and replies, "Your treat huh?" grinning slyly. "Yes, let's get some dope, can you score, I trashed all my dealer's numbers – Looks like you may know someone".

From there Jason didn't only relapse, but he actually used a needle for I.V. injection for the first time ever. In the moment, with an attractive girl, and a mind flooded with cravings that he thought were gone, he picked up the needle ready for a new experience. Before that, he had only snorted the drug. That night would be Jason's first and last genuine N.A. meeting. He not only started using the drug in a much more dangerous manner, but also unknowingly exposed himself to HIV, which he didn't know Jennifer already had. In his ignorance and enthusiasm for a fix – 2 months after being clean – he not only relapsed deeper into addiction than ever before, but also contracted a life threatening disease. He and Jennifer continued to go to N.A. together for a few more weeks before Jason stopped.

He was arrested for possession and paraphernalia. Jennifer continues to go, and is about to celebrate her 120 days clean from drugs. Nobody seems to confront Jennifer about using, and although she is not usually blatantly high like the night she met Jason, there are subtle clues that go unquestioned, such as long sleeve shirts on hot summer days to hide track marks and the occasional opiate induced scratching. The group is very proud of her, and she continues to wear her 4-month bracelet with pride – in overwhelming denial.

This may be an extreme example, but the fact that it is even *possible at all* makes it too real for comfort. I imagine you probably feel the same way when you really consider it. All too often, what happens when an A.A. or N.A. meeting fails is that they end up on some variety of maintenance drugs like methadone or Suboxone. These drugs are HIGHLY addictive and only worsen the toxic exposure. The longer one has fed the beast of addiction, the more the toxins get soaked up into the body.

Around in Circles – How to Say Out of the Spin-Zone

Can you see the terrible pattern here? Addicts often go from one method of treatment to the next, not even noticing that while each may appear uniquely different the hidden basic flaws in each are the same. They come to expect that after treatment relapse is to be expected and is 'normal'.

Hypothetical Jason has just started a circular process. Beginning with Inpatient, he seems successful for a few months. He just has to fight off some cravings from time to time. Then trying another method to curb his cravings to use, he attends N.A. During his time at N.A. he finds Jennifer and starts with the needle causing a full relapse. Next thing you know is he is arrested.

On getting out, once again 'sober', when the cravings start again he may decide to try maintenance therapy at a Methadone Clinic believing that this is not 'really' going back to drugs. Instantly, he loses what little sobriety he gained during incarceration by again introducing a new drug into his body and adding more toxins.

He may even try to detox from the methadone one day, upon realizing he is still a slave to an opiate, and simply receiving a **legal fix**. Now he has come full circle and is considering an inpatient center to get clean from the methadone treatment. Exactly where he started several years prior.

This is where Jason, through the encouragement and motivation of a family member, such as his mother or brother, has the chance to escape the circle of treatment centers.

By going through the Narconon program and receiving a proper detox, he won't have the lingering toxins making him so incredibly susceptible to relapse. As a student he will participate in his detox, according to a strict and proven method to remove the toxins through an exact combination of techniques based on both direct observation and a long history of success.

He will also, after completing a proper, active detox, enter phase two and learn life skills that he never knew existed. He will be able to use these new life shaping skills not only to stay drug free but also to succeed in his chosen vocation.

While this is a life changing experience it is not to be confused with any type of change in personality and character – it only takes his essence, and gives it newfound confidence and strength. Once he is *ready*, however long that may take, he will graduate as a successful student who has actively removed the relapse triggering toxins that no other program addresses. He will also have acquired a new attitude to life with a return of his native self-image and self-respect that he lost during his transgressions while using.

The staff will also be comfortable that Jason will not be a walking relapse waiting to happen when he leaves the program. This potential is real, and is entirely unique to the Narconon program, which has the lowest relapse rate of any program.

Or, there is another option for Jason...

Perhaps he can attempt to stop taking the methadone at a different, inpatient facility, if he can find another one, perhaps a better one than before?

Again, **perhaps** – and to that I would say, **perhaps = likely.**

Perhaps the 'new better' rehab will lead back to the N.A. meetings again. Perhaps he sticks with N.A. for a month or a year – he's doing so well, right? Well, perhaps one day a new, attractive girl, with pinprick pupils, and a slight itch starts him back all over again.

Without a proper detox behind him he is not strong enough to handle the temptation, not of flesh, but of the devil that sits upon the stoned girl's shoulders – mocking him, luring him to have another taste. The toxins are released, and the need to use is immediate.

Jason becomes an active user again. Whether he will continue the circle, go to prison for more crimes, or end up dead from an overdose are all possible outcomes when an addict follows these circles of varying, but basically the same ineffective treatments. The time between each "perhaps" can make this roundabout seem less obvious, especially to the addict, who is blinded by his own addiction and therefore cannot see it at all.

The good news is that this circle can be broken, but an even BETTER thing would be to go with what works first, and thus avoid the recycling treatments and relapses that are going to unfold. Some of your loved ones may have entered the circle, but it's imperative to know that it's not too late to escape it.

Those who are considering their first treatment program for their loved one should consider giving them the best chance of success from the beginning. This will save countless amounts of financial and emotional loss. With the right program the emotions can be repaired, but the money lost through funding useless treatments, methadone clinics, doctor's visits, medications, stolen money, treasured items pawned, and credit even ruined in acts of desperation to feed the habit, is all gone forever.

The guilt can be removed; the love and trust rebuilt, and a new life without chemicals can be attained.

What counts is actually ending the circle of flawed treatment and relapse, or never entering it to begin with. The Narconon program is the only program I have found that can fully heal a drug

50

addicted person and equip them with superior life skills to prevent the fall back into the hole of addiction ever again.

6

Passive Detox vs. Active Detox

The detoxification period is the first of two important stages that a truly successful treatment program will provide. The second stage, which contains life changing, spiritual development techniques and strategies (not based on any specific denomination), will be discussed in chapter 9 under *Personal Enhancement.*

The detox stage is typically what your addicted loved one undoubtedly fears the most. The truth is, most addicts *really do* want to get clean and stay that way, but their drug of choice has conditioned them in many ways, consciously and subconsciously, to believe this is not possible.

So what are your loved ones so afraid of? It surely can't be that hard to stop, can it?

Well, unfortunately that depends on many factors, and the truth is this: by using the right treatment approach from the start, it really is easier to overcome than the addict imagines.

However, it is important to understand that to most addicts who have gone through a treatment program and then relapsed – as so many have – there is a sense of failure and guilt for not having succeeded. Never mind the money that was wasted. They develop a feeling of the impossibility of ever getting drug free. The addict comes to believe that sobriety is just not possible *for them,* despite any evidence you show them or stories you tell of other addicts' successes in getting off.

Of course this is a fallacy, and the drugs feed it, nourish it even. Think of the commonly used theme to represent conflicts in someone's consciousness, often depicted in films and cartoons: the angel on one shoulder, and the devil on the other. The angel provides the voice of reason, encouragement, hope, and an overall moral perspective that would lead the person in the right direction. Conversely, on the opposite shoulder is the devil. The devil encourages wrong behavior, an immoral lifestyle, lies, cheating, stealing, and anything to serve a selfish and self-centered motivation that lacks morality and promotes nothing but a thought process to justify these aforementioned flaws of character.

What does a metaphorical angel and devil on opposing shoulders have to do with the process of detoxification? Well, it is going to be different for each addict, depending on whether they have attempted a treatment regime before and failed, tried on their own and failed, or never tried at all – fearing failure is natural enough. In every one of these situations, as the power of the drugs take affect the angel perched on your loved ones shoulders will slowly but surely start to fade away.

This is the worst scenario, because as the voice of hope and reason begins to fade, the opposite voice of the metaphoric devil continually gets louder, stronger, and takes more control.

Now, I'm certainly speaking in a metaphoric sense, but the application itself is very real: your loved one, the person you knew and have supported unconditionally, despite hardships IS the angel. Even during their drug use, they will initially maintain a semblance of themselves – the angel is still on their shoulder, and although they may not listen to her, she is there nevertheless trying to talk away the devil and regain control. Unfortunately, the devil IS the drugs or alcohol, and this particular battle between good and evil, the devil will almost always win. It is extremely hard for anyone to remove the devil from their shoulders – or stop their drug intake – on their own. Drugs offer a false sense of comfort, and the person has to re-learn how to find comfort in life without them, something that was so easy before they started.

Removing the drugs and their influence on the person is obviously something that only the experts of *successful* rehabilitation centers can do. The first step is to detoxify from the drug.

Only when the drugs have been eliminated can the treatment program teach your loved ones, as a student, how to become themselves again and acquire the skills and strength they need to live drug free. Skills that were missing that made them susceptible to taking drugs in the first place.

As it turns out this is very possible, but it can only be achieved using the right method - which brings me to the point of detoxification itself. There are two types of detox that exist, but are rarely differentiated: active detox which *is* successful, and the passive forms of detox, which are bound to result in a re-emergence of the old drug influence. Let me explain what a passive detox involves – or more accurately lacks. From there, I'll explain what an active detox does, and how it is without question the only method that works every time to rid these drugs from the person's body.

The Passive Detox and the Tragedy Thereof

As already noted, your loved one is inevitably afraid of detoxing. This fear is the drug speaking. The drugs are in control of their behavior and actions. Full detox removes that.

Now, when a person is dependent on drugs, the thought of doing a detox is usually uncomfortable physically and mentally. This is a good thing, believe it or not.

A passive detox, however, only *hides* the drug effects and even the doctors, counselors, and psychiatrists cannot see that the drug influence is still there lurking in the metabolites and will continue to linger for years if not removed. A passive detox does not address the drug metabolites that are still hanging around, waiting to re-emerge. This emergence may happen immediately after treatment even if the treatment center says the detox is complete.

Countless addicts who have gone through passive detoxifications will readily admit that even while they were still in treatment, they already had intentions to use again as soon as the clock ran out – simply going through the motions, telling the doctors and counselors what they wanted to hear, in eager anticipation of the day they were let out the door and back into the world.

This is an extreme example of how powerful the drugs and the lingering metabolites are, and certainly some people may last for months, or even years without using – but with the drug metabolites still lingering inside, all it takes is a tiny release of these metabolites (often during stressful situations or strenuous activities) and here come the cravings and soon after that it's back to using again. This may happen after a month or after several years, but the usual and unfortunate reality is that it *will* happen.

Additionally, if a treatment center only does this kind of incomplete detox and then over the top of that attempts to get the person to engage in some sort of life changing strategies and philosophies to prepare them for a new life that will NOT work either. The metabolites will come back to beat them in the end.

To win this part of the battle you need to provide an active detox AND a battery of well tested successful life changing strategies. Only offering one or the other does not work long term. While either one may win the battle of the moment they

57

will not win the war. A treatment center needs to get *both* parts done properly. Half way there is not enough and is why a program must use an active detox approach before the emotional or spiritual phase.

Before explaining how the active detox works and why it is superior and necessary for any other action to work, I'm going to explain what a passive detox approach is, and why it fails... again and again.

All this mention of 'passive detox' may seem strange. You may be thinking, "But what is passive about the facility that used medicine to wean my loved one down from his drug of choice?" Or maybe, "I tried helping my son detox at home, he was a wreck and stayed in bed, so I 'actively' took care of him and gave him the time he needed to sober-up, making sure he had someone to cook for him and look after him." Believe me I sympathize with those who have tried this method. Their intentions are very worthwhile and I have heard similar statements many times before from family members trying to keep their loved ones 'comfortable' during an emotionally straining time (either with home care or medication administering inpatient centers) – *but* such conversations arise out of desperation, frustration, and an inability to understand why their loved ones did, in fact, go on to relapse. It is also the point in such conversations in which I relate the difference between these passive approaches that *seem* active, but in reality, are not.

The first issue to be addressed is that medical detox is not an active detox at all. It is simply introducing more medications, which such centers often like to label as "comfort meds". These meds are reduced extremely slowly so that the addict does not go through withdrawal as severely. The problem here is that more medications are not only introducing more toxins into the body, but also providing a false sense of 'ease' to the addict. There is no 'free lunch', so-to-speak when coming off hard drugs or alcohol. Your loved one needs to actually experience their detox, be a part of the detox and actually "own" their detox. To numb the process with medication is not really doing the process at all.

I actually hesitate to even give such programs the credit of the word 'detox' itself, as there is nothing that is done to remove the drug toxins at all. All they are doing is adding more drugs until the patient slowly *by their standards* starts to "appear normal' again.

This is an enormous illusion because the drug use is not stopping; it's just being regulated by the center as if it was a food diet! Yes, there are healthier ways to eat, and replacing greasy French fries with a salad is a healthy choice. The thing is, there are *not* healthier ways to use drugs, and a medicated detox implies that this is the case. This actually makes the detox 'seem' to work smoothly, because once the medications are stopped completely (if they ever are) the withdrawal might appear to be easier than they have experienced in the past. This is not an achievement; it is a step backwards when one needs to move forward. It also will make a relapse much more likely because there are now more new toxins left behind from the "comfort meds".

The addict will think, "That wasn't so bad after all, I can probably use again once in a while and not get a problem. Besides, even if I do, which I won't (false security) that was a breeze – I can "detox" anytime!" This is why the typical scenario after a medicated detox is a relapse. Do you want this revolving door kind of treatment center, where your loved one will be going in and out and in and out for years and years to come? Is this really the one you want to choose?

If you don't want this kind of rehab roundabout, then maybe your loved one or you yourself may feel attracted to what must be the worst possible choice, a maintenance program, such as methadone. This, when it comes right down to it, is no more than swapping one addictive drug for another addictive drug.

Then there are inpatient programs that offer a 'dry out' detox – which is only a very, very slight improvement upon the medicated detox. The 'home detox' is essentially the same as any inpatient center that does non-medicated dry-outs. Both leave the addict alone expecting and hoping them to 'wait-out' the physical withdrawal and cravings.

Do you honestly think this is going to achieve anything long term?

Considering that this is supposed to be the "turning point" for inpatient centers which can cost thousands of dollars for no more than a ticking clock, it's really sad that someone could actually get talked into paying for it.

The story pretty much goes like this: Go to bed, kick around a bit, times up, and then off you go – to relapse, of course. Because nothing is done to actively address the fact that just because an addict has gone to bed and is now out of bed after a week or so it doesn't mean he or she is not still LOADED with drugs and metabolite toxins.

We still have the condition we started with and in particular the metabolites that cause all the trouble are still in the fat where they *will* stay – unless of course, they are removed. Wait a minute... removed? You may be thinking, "I've been hearing all the horrors of how there appears to be *nothing* that can be done and I now realize that the drug metabolites stay in the body, stuck in the fatty tissue, what I want to know is, is there is a way to **remove them?**"

Yes there is, and stressing that most rehabilitation centers do not understand this crucial fact, it is important to fully understand the reason why a true **active detox** is the **only way** to get sober and not walk away from the detox still full of these crave-causing metabolites.

61

7

The Active Detox – Why it is Essential for Lasting Rehabilitation

So far, I've gone to great lengths to expose the problems of the many forms and varieties of what I am calling the passive detox models – some, such as methadone do not even qualify as detox, but rather a **legal fix** or you might say, **retox** (a word you won't find in any dictionary, unfortunately, but used for representing the *addition*, rather than *subtraction* of poisonous, toxic, drugs and their lasting metabolites), and are really a counter-productive treatment.

Now, it is time to introduce the model of an active detoxification program, where you can understand with clarity the huge differences. I want to explain why such a model is truly the only way to give your loved one the gift of completely removing not only the easily available drugs lodged in their body but also the (otherwise) everlasting toxins that are buried beneath the surface, so to speak.

But let me pause for a moment and answer this common question that gets asked all the time. It is one that continues to bother me the more I read about, witness, and personally watch the circular pattern of the treatment 'attempts' that fail again and again.

The question is:
 If the Narconon method is so successful in removing ALL the drugs and their residues from the person's body, why don't other treatment centers use the same proven method to remove these toxins?

That is a very good question, and even after painstaking, unbiased research I have not found any *good* reasons for this unforgivable flaw that thrives throughout the majority of the addiction treatment industry. I have my suspicions, and most of them can be observed and described in one word: money.

If you have a guaranteed repeat business model as is the case with these revolving door programs there is simply no incentive to solve the problem.

There is also the Authority factor. People claiming to be an authority dig in if they consider that their position is being challenged. Rather than being open to new ideas, if they didn't think of it first, they reject out of hand any new ideas. As an authority they believe they have to be the source of all developments in their subject. No one is allowed to think outside their square. It gets worse. If some new research does show up that is outside their fundamental beliefs, they attack it with ferocity because they feel it threatens their position, their existence -- and even more so if it threatens their livelihood.

For instance, the authoritarian groups that run the medical model believe that people are made up of nothing more than chemicals. There is no actual *person* present beyond their brain. Now we don't have to get into that argument and it doesn't really matter for the moment. Personally I find it insulting, but I only mention it to explain what the medical/psychiatric model people use as a base for all their "research". It's true. This concept is the fundamental on which all their work is based. People are nothing more than brains.

So from this unproven belief, they claim that anything that goes "wrong" is only a problem in chemistry. This concept of course restricts them to the use of chemicals as the only method or resource they can use to treat anything.

Therefore the only thing that they can to do when addressing a "person's" problem is to muck about with their chemistry. In fact as far as they are concerned the "reason" someone is an addict or anything else they might suffer from is still only a problem in chemistry. Get the chemicals right or "balanced" and all will be well.

They absolutely believe that all behavior and anything else to do with a human being is nothing more than chemicals interacting in the brain. No different from the circuits in a robot or a recipe for a cake or an atom bomb. I have actually asked these people to show me the integrity molecule, the honesty synapse, the art atom or the chemical formula the brain uses for composing music. The answers I have been given are certainly amusing as they defy any reason.

Anyway, when applying this chemical theory fails to get the person off drugs and fails everywhere else where they label people's difficulties as "diseases" such as ADHD and other "behavioral problems" they roll out the Gene theory. It's all in your genes they say, and nothing can be done about it anyway, but if you give us some more research funds we will do some chemical experiments and let you know what happens. The fact is this scam has been going on just far too long and its exposure as such is long overdue.

Now this is not to be confused with the genuine medical doctor with his prescription medicines long proven to counteract actual diseases like polio and snake bite and measles and the like where the virus or bacteria causing the trouble can be seen by anybody with a microscope. That's not the issue here. What is the issue is that no medical model rehab operator can show you the addiction bacteria, virus or gene and never will because that is not where the cause will be found. It also will not be found in the brain chemistry. Yes, the brain can be damaged by drugs. We know that from the basic definition of a drug. It is not a food. It is a poison. And that is chemistry, not a virus or bacteria. The only difference between the effect and the damage it does is in the amount of drug (poison) taken.

It must be remembered that the body is a self-perpetuating, self-repairing mechanism.

Despite what people do to it, its inbuilt mechanisms are programed for survival. That is its total goal. It is a goal it has always had. That goal is what has brought it to its present efficiency and development. It has been at it for a very long time. It knows instantly when it is fed something that is food. It knows instantly when it is fed something that is not food or is a poison. When purposely fed poison it will use all its inbuilt mechanisms to protect itself and try to reject or neutralize the poison one way or the other. It can only do this up to a point before it goes into overload. These are the three stages of drug intake. Remember, first it gets a boost, a high, as it goes into action to combat the poison. Then it gets drowsy and it puts the person to sleep while it uses every bit of its energy to neutralize the poison. If this defensive action fails and the drugging continues it goes into complete overload and succumbs to the poison. As you can see, although deadly, it is not a complicated process.

Understanding this simple process one would surely have to wonder why anyone would ever even consider or suggest using drugs to treat drug addicts.

Drugs, or you might as well say, poisons, are already the problem. The body in its natural effort to survive when under the onslaught of drugs does not suddenly produce a neutralizing drug to combat the poison. So again, the idea of giving it yet another drug to handle drug addiction is already a completely unnatural approach.

What the drug addicted person needs first of all is a procedure to get the existing drugs completely out of the body. That's what is causing the person distress right now, an overdose of drugs. Not some unknown bacteria or gene or brain imbalance, it's just being poisoned beyond its ability to survive. You can't do any more for a person's ability to reason and take responsibility until that is handled. There is no point in trying to do anything else for the person until this immediate condition of drug overload is handled.

This stunt of **falsely** labeling addiction as an incurable disease actually does serve a purpose: It gives the medical model supporters something to say when faced with a genuine successful rehabilitation from alternative programs. What they say is, "The 'disease' is only in remission, and thus susceptible to re-emerging". They use this excuse to explain their own relapses, i.e. the "disease" came back.

For the majority of addicts, relapse is a sad and unfortunate reality. The medical and academic population then retort, "Yes, the disease is back, remember we said it was incurable after all". So, it seems that the medical/academic community, can't provide any solutions, has plenty of excuses, offers no emotional or spiritual reconciliation, and has nothing really effective to offer. All you get is a walking, talking relapse waiting to happen. Remember the question I posed at the beginning: Do I get results or do I get excuses?

Hostile? Yes, but it is very much a justified hostility. Why is that? Well, for myself and for parents, friends, and family members who have been through the rollercoaster ride of ups and downs (and likely still are at this moment), going through the repeating pattern of: addiction, jails, weeks without using, relapses, meetings, inpatient, outpatient, meetings, maintenance therapy, detox, meetings, inpatient, relapse, outpatient, meetings, detox, relapse, prison, detox, weeks without using, another week without using, a year without, 5 years without, FINALLY starting to regain hope, relapse, meetings, inpatient, longer prison sentences, outpatient, maintenance, weeks without using, relapse...

Hostility at this system that is so prevalent – certainly.

Yes, the order and extent of the routine outlined above will be different for each person, but without **stopping** the vicious, and seemingly endless cycle that is far more painful in reality than on paper, you and your loved one's life will just be a sad variation of the above. It won't be just words to you; it will be a collection of haunting experiences that leave you stressed, frustrated and with a feeling of hopelessness.

The thing is; there IS hope. There IS a solution. No matter how many failures your loved one has undergone, the solution is in doing a full **active detoxification** which removes all the drugs and their associated lingering metabolites from their body. When this is followed with a life-changing rehabilitation section as discussed in Phase 2 the person does become drug free for life.

8

Active Detoxification Explained

The Only Proven Way Out of the Treatment Circle

If I asked an audience of family members or anyone who had an addicted loved one, "How long they would expect their sobriety to last?" I would have a very puzzled and confused audience – "Forever", "Indefinitely", "The rest of her life" would be the unanimous answer and they would wonder why I would even ask such a question.

If you ask some rehabs this same question you should get the same answer. Far too many will not give you a definitive answer.

The question then becomes, why can't you tell me?

Of course they can't tell you because they don't have a rehab that achieves that as a normal predictable final result of doing their program. If it does happen at all it is because of the patient's absolute determination despite the program.

So what exactly *is* this active detox method?

The Basics of the Active Detox – The ONLY model known to end the Cycle of Relapse

The Narconon detoxification process doesn't advertise itself as an active detox program. In fact, that's a term I've actually coined for illustrative purposes to highlight the difference between this detox and its uniqueness to many others in general use. This point is so often overlooked and is the key to its success.

The fact is these lingering drug metabolites will not leave the fatty tissue by themselves. They have to be actively removed. This is done through a very precise planned routine of replacement oils. What happens is the new fresh oils are taken up by the fatty tissues and the fats containing the drug metabolites are released naturally and flushed out of the body. There is no way this can happen on its own. No "sitting in a sauna" for hours or doing sweat programs will shake them out. They have to be driven out by an exact routine.

They must be removed *during* the detoxification portion of the program; otherwise they will be released at a later time, during any strenuous or stressful activity – during a N.A. meeting perhaps – which will lead to a relapse. Although the example of temptation during Jason's N.A. meeting was fictitious, it is only a variation of what all too often happens. In fact, from my research it seems this is more the common way the cycle of addiction continues, not through any character flaw itself. After all Jason was well-intentioned, but because the residual toxins were still in his body ready to come out and start the cravings all over again leaving him as just another relapse waiting to happen.

PAWS

Is a funny term that medical professionals are now using to describe these cravings and the consequential relapses which occur at various times after their method of detox is said to be complete. The term is relatively new (within the last 5-10 years) as the PR lobbyists have realized that this relapse phenomenon is becoming too well noticed, so they have scrambled to place a name on it: Post-Acute Withdrawal Syndrome or PAWS.

The truth is there is no such thing as PAWS. It is simply an invention. A silly new PR name for relapse which has been happening all the time. If you don't get the drug metabolites out of the body you will later on get cravings which ends as a relapse. It is a simple as that. If you do the detox properly this doesn't happen.

So PAWS is only a name for not having properly flushed all the toxins (metabolites) from the body. That's all there is to that.

I believe that giving something a name for not having done your job properly which you can then use as an excuse to invent or administer even more toxic drugs shows the heartless arrogance of these operators.

73

I guess their plan is that if you put a fancy sounding name on it people will accept that it is sort of normal and to be expected. People might even believe you know what you are doing. You can also claim that you are working on a new wonder drug solution for it thus diverting attention off the fact that your treatment failed.

So, the next time you hear the mention of PAWS, this is what is *actually* happening to the person, and likely has already happened to your loved ones many, many times if they have relapsed. In their denial of these phenomena the best the medical model community can do is to give this craving and relapse recurring routine a silly name, say it is to be expected, say there's nothing you can do about it or say they are searching for yet another new drug to prescribe to counteract it.

Anyway, in my view, this simply proves that the medical and academic communities have no place in addiction treatment, because there is no real desire or motivation for them to find a cure. Fortunately, for those who see though this, which might be difficult at first, given the sheer power of such institutions and their advertising budget, there is hope. That hope is found in the Narconon detoxification process by using the following techniques. Only then can true recovery at the personal level ever be achieved.

So, what are the key points in an active detox program?

The Narconon Detox – How and Why it Works

Let's quickly go through the facts again so the whole drug cycle is clear.

1 – Drugs are basically poisons, No drug has any food component or food value.

2 – Metabolism is the process by which the body turns food into energy

3 – Drugs are oil soluble, they mix with fat. They are not water soluble.

4 – When drugs enter the system digestion begins and the body tries to dissolve the chemical.

5 - The blood and body fluids are water soluble. These separate from the drug.

6 – As the drugs pass through the system they don't all get dissolved by digestion or fully excreted, but being oil based bits of them (metabolites) get attracted to and lodge in the fatty tissues.

7 – They can stay lodged in these fatty tissues for years.

8-- During periods of high activity or stress, a little of these residual toxins (metabolites) will leak from the fatty tissue back into the bloodstream.

9 – Now active in the system, these metabolites will cause the person to actually taste the original drug again and this is the cause of craving.

10 – Now, having returned to the same state they were in during active drug use, not only is a relapse to be expected, it is almost unavoidable.

Removing and Replacing Toxins
Out with the Bad In with the Good

Narconon has researched and developed an effective, medically safe, and most importantly, a consistent working model for detoxification from any and every drug. While simple, it is detailed, and very specific. This is important when it comes to the removal of the residual toxins left in the fatty tissues. For the personal comfort of the person doing this process they need to be flushed out as quickly and efficiently as possible. The method used to remove these toxins is quite powerful, so there must be an intake of healthy, natural vitamins, minerals, good food and water to counter-balance this flushing out process. Don't confuse a safe, active detox, with any medical model of treatment however. The way in which toxins are removed is rigorous, as it must be, but also safe – so basic, fundamental medical care is taken into account. Otherwise, issues such as dehydration or nutritional problems may arise. Narconon is aware of such possibilities, and as such, monitors the physical condition of its students undergoing the detoxification phase. This phase needs to be fully completed before any real learning experiences can begin. While these toxins are still in the body and brain, the drugs are still controlling the person. Concentration, focus, as well as clear rational thinking is difficult if not impossible.

Metabolite Removal

Essentially, toxins are removed via an exchange process. They are removed by replacing the contaminated fat in the fatty tissue with new fresh clean fat.

To make this exchange happen the person does a regimen of low heat sauna to promote sweating, exercise to increase the metabolic rate, a diet full of fiber rich high quality food and plenty of vegetables to promote healthy and frequent bowel movements, a strict and specific measured intake of essential vitamins and minerals to replenish anything that might be lost during the exchange process and of course a healthy intake of water to ensure that dehydration does not occur.

Because drugs are a fat based substance the metabolites of them get attracted to the fatty tissue like a magnet. When the body is fed a measured and controlled dose of the right kind of edible oil (a fat based substance) it has been discovered that the body will release the existing fat from these tissues and take up this new oil and turn it into the fat it needs.

77

As this takes place the old toxin loaded fat is released and replaced with this fresh new clean fat, thereby "flushing out" these drug metabolites.

This action cleans the body of all drug residues.

With the metabolites gone the body is now finally truly clean.

This means that later on when the person is engaging in strenuous exercise or under stress or otherwise sweating there are no drug residues to excrete into the bloodstream to cause craving along with the virtually guaranteed consequence of relapse. It is this action that ends the cycle of the revolving door and the endless failures rife in other programs.

Medical supervision is only in place to ensure safety during the detox stage. It is not there to implement any 'medical model' ideology. The medical staffs for Narconon detox are there simply to ensure that students undergoing the process remain medically sound.

This needs to be stressed, because some may worry about their loved ones undergoing what can sound like a rigorous detox, fearing that health may be compromised. Such worries can certainly be put to rest, as Narconon treats safety and well-being as a top priority for all of its students.

The word *clean* is used very often when speaking about drug use. I think this is a very good term, but unfortunately poorly understood. Not using drugs alone will never get a person

78

clean. Only with an active detox program, where you exercise, sweat, eat healthy, drink plenty of water, and do the fat exchange part will you actually scrub a person's fatty tissue clean. When used to describe a person who is not currently using, but still has the drug residuals sitting in their fat, well that's like claiming a person is 'clean' because they put on perfume or cologne. Sure, they may *seem* to smell nice and fresh, but underneath the façade is a body that is dirty, unwashed, and unkempt

The only way to really get clean is to actually take the time to get in the bath, so-to-speak, and start scrubbing away the dirt. Only an active detox program in the fullest sense of the words achieves that.

9

After Detoxification – Phase Two

The Personal Enhancement Phase

Once a student has completed the detoxification phase and removed the drug toxins they are ready to re-enter the world again, right? Well, not quite. The detox is certainly the most important first-step towards achieving any hope of lasting sobriety, but that is not enough alone. That only handles the physical side. Now they need to address the remaining factors that allowed them to fall by the wayside in the first place as well as build up their confidence and strength so they don't fall again.

Mental recovery is an entirely personal process, and almost impossible to achieve without help and direction from those with actual knowledge and understanding of the key principles involved. This key action is not available in the standard medical model. The façade of counseling, whether individual or group, suggests that this is taking place in the average 30, 60, or 90 day program. However, it is not. Instead a dialogue of absolutely no value continues over and over again – goals are not developed, and underlying problems are not resolved.

Counseling or consultation becomes no more than simply a person venting random experiences to a listener who often really does care but who has no correct knowledge or the kind of skills needed to relieve the person of their difficulties. At the end of the sitting the person is no different and no better than they were at the start. They may experience some relief as it always helps to tell someone your troubles but apart from that nothing else is achieved. In fact what they usually get is a bombardment of evaluation and advice. Nothing is done to actually relieve the emotional backlog or the personal hang-ups.

Valuable time and energy is simply wasted - which is not only astonishing when you really think about it, but also leaves the painful memories of guilt, hopelessness, despair and boredom to remain as hang-ups in the addicts mind. *This* is the type of thinking that needs to be addressed, as that is what keeps the person pinned to the past. By leaving the person's mind attached to the past, they are trapped and can never freely move on from these mental blocks and achieve a *change of attitude and heart*, which is what they actually need to do.

Do you believe in miracles? The Narconon graduates certainly do, because they say that's what they experience on this part of the program. While Narconon's statistics are evidence of this happening, to fully appreciate it, it must be experienced. What you are witnessing at a graduation is *life* rehabilitation, not just 'drug' rehabilitation.

It is in this life changing, attitude changing and personal enhancement phase of the program where the past, the present, and the future of the student is handled. In this phase your loved one will experience *clean* in the true sense of the word. Clean, inside and out. The body, having been washed clean of the drug toxins, and the spirit or personality also made clean, fully replenished, nurtured, and ready to take on the world anew. Here is where the students become entirely new versions of themselves, everything that they were before they started using is there, but now they have the confidence, skills, and peace of mind knowing that they are truly clean – success is not just a hope, it is a certainty. In this sense, they may finally be honestly clean for the first time ever. From the first hit of a joint, the first line of cocaine, the first shot of whiskey, the first shot of heroin – it was all lingering in every single Narconon student when they first walked in the door.

Walking out, they have been completely restored to their old self again, but now stronger willed and more able to live a sober clean life than ever before. Seeing the transformation is amazing, and perhaps that's why doctors are slow – but starting to come around – to give the Narconon program the obvious merit that it deserves. The results, when viewed from their perspective, are nothing short of miracles. I know this is not any 'miracle' at work, but rather a highly effective, rehabilitation method taking place, as can be seen in its graduates.

Life Skills and Cleaning up Past Misdeeds

Part of this second phase is a comprehensive activity to help students learn how to live their lives without once again succumbing to addiction or needing illicit drugs, or alcohol, if that was the addiction.

How this is accomplished is paradoxically simple, yet also extremely detailed and absolutely necessary. This is the stage of the program in which students learn new life-changing skills and how to develop a new way of dealing with the problems and hardships in life, including the issues that brought about their initial use of drugs.

There is no way to actually write how this learning process happens completely, as it is individually tailored to each student. The big difference is that although there is certainly a proven successful curriculum, applicable to *all* Narconon students, it also *must* be used and applied to each individual student. This is another aspect that other treatment programs simply do not understand when employing a 'catch-all' counseling approach.

The procedure here is one of cognitive learning where the person gains new understandings about how they see things.

This all-in-together method has been proven not to work. Even though everyone who experiences drug addiction certainly has gone through similar things in life, the way in which they actually came to these similarities will be different for each person.

Students must learn to look to their own unique past and face up to all the pain and suffering they caused not only to themselves, but also their family, friends, significant others, etc.

First of all they get to learn how to comfortably face other people again. Yes, amazingly, this is something they have forgotten how to do or never learned in the first place. Deep down they are actually hiding as they know very well the things they have done were harmful.

These actions are called non-survival actions rather than moral transgressions because they more accurately describe what they are doing. Morals tend to have religious connotations and this is not a religious issue as such. Taking stuff that isn't yours to take from friends or strangers without their permission is plainly not a survival action. While the addict might believe it helps his survival for the moment in some drug twisted mind computation it sure doesn't do much for the survival of the person being stolen from. Reducing the body's ability to live by poisoning it with drugs is a non-survival act.

It is a fact that when a person does things that are illegal or harmful they withdraw from the area or person they have harmed. Technically, it's called, "going out of communication". This has to be repaired. You can't have a one sided conversation. You can't have a conversation with someone who won't reply.

The students do little exercises that handle this "out of communication" condition that bring them back into communication with those around them.

Then there is the cleaning up of the past actions.

With the materials to hand in this phase they come to understand what made them an addict, how their situation came to be, and how they now have a chance to finally get control of their lives and move ahead without being tied to any guilt or shame from their past actions.

Students are opened up to a non-judgmental and confidential action, totally unique to Narconon which allows them to face their past without any reservations and to take full responsibility for their earlier activities.

This action frees them from their past non-survival (harmful to self and others) actions and allows them to repair all the damage they have done to their friends, family, others and even themselves. This section is where they say miracles take place. The relief and excitement to be seen in a student's eyes when they complete this action and can again genuinely hug someone they love with a clear heart and conscience is a magical moment to behold.

With all this over and out of the way the student then looks to their future. They have a look at the common rules that we all live under. They set their future goals and make plans for where they go from here. This is a very exciting phase where they *know* they are drug free for life and can make plans with great confidence. At this point they are ready to graduate as a clean drug free person with an active, productive, even creative and certainly decent life ahead of them.

Many say it's like having a second chance but better because they are now armed with the knowledge they desperately needed before they started taking drugs as a solution to whatever it was worrying them at the time.

The graduation ceremony is an experience to witness. To hear graduates talk of their trials and tribulations going through the program - and believe me there are plenty of those - is nothing short of amazing.

Getting drug free can be pretty dramatic at times. The staff has seen it all before of course, many are ex-addicts themselves, which makes them eminently capable of helping the student through the rough bits with total understanding of what the student is going through.

It is a hard heart that can remain unmoved at a graduation. Watching families being re-united, sons, daughters and spouses with eyes now clear and sparkling again, hugs all around. The excited chatter about the changes they have experienced. The wins they have had on the program. The buzz of re-vitalized dreams and of future plans. I must say, at a graduation it is often hard to find a dry eye.

10

My Purpose

The world can't help but notice, sometimes with envy, what it may not yet understand.

There is also the fact that the world is made up of two kinds of people. There are those who try to make things better for themselves and others, and those who get pleasure in making things worse. This is observable in all walks of life regardless of the clothes they wear or the position they hold in society. Sometimes one has to be a bit stern to get things done but that is not the same as creating havoc and unhappiness all around.

As far as I am concerned the people who make and push addictive drugs fall into the latter category. Anyone who seduces another or others into drug addiction is not your friend. The untold destruction drugs cause in people's lives is not the result of a friendly act. An organization that dispenses drugs as a solution to drugs is of similar ilk.

Those who attack people of goodwill who actually can and do make things better for others are about as despicable as you can get.

When people of this type get into positions of power and authority we have a very dangerous situation. As history has shown, they send otherwise friendly, innocent young men to war to kill other innocent friendly young men. These types of people can appear very friendly. Hitler was a very popular man with the soldiers he was training to be killers.

Drugs and drug addiction is the scourge of modern society. It is a very lucrative business.

Its solution, I believe will be in education. If kids and people in general had the whole picture of what drugs do *and* had better alternative solutions to their everyday problems and worries they would never ever even remotely consider drowning their sorrows in drugs.

As far as 'recreational' drugs are concerned that is just another trick name put about by the pushers playing on people's desire to feel happy and forget about their worries. In that very statement is the answer to drugs. Why are they not already happy? What is stopping them being happy as they are?

Have you ever watched little kids playing and having a great time? Do they need drugs to be that way? Of course not. Would drugs make them any happier? Of course not. You will never see unhappy adults made that happy no matter how many drugs they take. So drugs are obviously not the way to happiness. All they ever do is dumb the person down so they don't notice so much the other things that are on their mind. If they can't be happy naturally that itself is a problem.

So my claim remains. Until people find better alternatives to handle their everyday worries and concerns or find ways to let their natural happiness shine through, those people are easy prey to drug pushers. Until people make progress in that direction we will be saddled with addiction.

In the meantime we need a way to get people off who have been caught up in the scourge. A way that not only ends addiction permanently but also puts them beyond the reach of pushers for the rest of their life because they now have better solutions to the worries of everyday life and a superior knowledge about the subject. In other words, a way to be happy and successful without drugs.

Part of my goal in writing this book – perhaps my greatest aspiration, even - is to spread this message, so more people are able to finally understand there *is* a cure to addiction. There is no disease in your loved ones life related to their use of drugs, so using the word 'cure' may seem paradoxical, but it is a helpful figure of speech in this sense, and not meant to imply any illness was ever present. Perhaps poor judgment is as far as it goes, but to consider poor judgment itself a disease, well then I'd imagine we have all had moments of that disease, and as pointed out earlier, it is only a figure of speech.

I encourage you to look past the deception, and the sweet talk you see in the advertisements

91

and the commercials put out by drug rehabs that are using drugs to treat drugs. These operations are essentially just another business. Something that, sadly, drug addiction treatment has become. Let that sink in for a moment... because it's imperative to understand and see through the PR you will inevitably come across. Businesses are developed to make money. If overcoming addiction wasn't profitable, you wouldn't see so many operators in the business with so many different options offering to overcome your loved ones terrible condition.

Doing this research was a huge eye opener for me and I hope I can save you a lot of wasted time and heartbreak by making this information available to you in this small book.

Time may not be on your side. There is no time to waste when lives could be at stake. There is no point in waiting on the next trend in treatment or some new wonder drug. None of that is going to change anything.

The fact is, so long as they are using drugs or abusing alcohol, they are not living, they are simply receiving credit for being alive – there's a big difference. What you don't need is for that credit to run out and you lose them altogether.

Broken Promises
Now we come to a very important point I must make.
There is also no point in listening to your loved one's endless stories and promises about

how they are going to change their ways. How tomorrow they will stop using. How they will never steal or pawn your treasured valuables again. These are empty promises to get you to leave them alone. To keep things just as they are so they can avoid facing up to the situation they are in. Do not make the mistake of believing what they say. They will say anything that they think will keep you happy and off their back. If this is going on it becomes your integrity that is now under threat. Believing their stories or their promises makes you a party to their addiction. By not taking action you are actually condoning what they are doing. Truly loving them is doing something to break them out of their addiction. Agreeing with them will never do that. Remember you are not talking to your loved one at all. You are talking to a drug affected mind. You are only talking to drugs.

They don't call them mind altering drugs for nothing. You are being manipulated just as they are by their drug affected mind. I am sure you have already found that out. You see their real problem, never announced, is what led them into taking drugs in the first place. The problem they thought they couldn't face or couldn't handle. They will never tell you what that is. In fact, I have discovered that this only comes to light in the second phase of the Narconon program when they are clean enough in body and strong enough in mind to face it. Until they have gone through withdrawal, detox, and some of phase 2 they are not responsible enough to discuss rationally what made them turn to drugs or do they have the mental strength to do anything about it even if they did.

In the meantime do not believe their stories. They are all excuses to avoid facing the situation they are currently in.

I cannot overstate my encouragement and enthusiasm for the Narconon program. It is the only program that I know to exist, that actually gets people clean, in the real sense of the word as it applies to addiction. I would gladly support any other program that follows in a similar fashion, should one exist, but currently I have not found any others that actually do work this consistently.

You may get lucky with some other program, or hear stories of people who have gotten off, but without an active detox I can tell you now, based on these discoveries, that their body is still not truly clean.

The frightening difference today is that more people are using drugs than ever, and it has now become an attractive business model simply taking money from caring parents or friends, who are desperate to save a loved one's life. That difference is important, because as addiction treatment becomes more of a commodity then the ethics of running one could soon vanish completely. I hope you have the chance to read this before that happens.

The fact is, Narconon invests all its effort into making people drug free and otherwise saving lives. As a not-for-profit organization it doesn't have the profit surplus or government subsidies to spend copious dollars on advertising. No, they are too busy ending addiction.

With the industry becoming a profit motivated operation, ending addiction permanently would be bad for business. The last thing they want is people who are 'cured'. They won't be returning again, and again, for more of the same ineffective treatment. Threatened, as they feel, from a program that works, they spend money that should be used to make their model actually work on attacking Narconon through shameless PR stunts and false claims. They see it as a threat to their business model.

Think of the political advertisements you see in print and on television, and how they always try to either promote themselves beyond what is true, or attack their opponent to make them appear to be a bad choice. Narconon suffers its share of this spin doctor type of mudslinging nonsense.

The truth will always eventually show itself, and I'm here to help speed that process so you won't have to wait for that happenstance moment when maybe one day you bump into a Narconon graduate before you get to hear the amazing Narconon success story.

Now that I know the Narconon story for what it really is I feel a moral obligation to do my part as a writer, and pass this knowledge on. I have personally watched too many people who I love, fall into the trap of ineffective treatment centers and the subsequent relapses.

I want to put before you this option, and give you a chance to think critically 'outside the box', which will help lead you and your loved ones out of the terrible circle of addiction.

If you have a drug addiction problem you need to give Narconon a call. You can ask to speak to former graduates if you like. They are always more than happy to answer any questions from a concerned family member, friend, or spouse who is caught up in the drug trap.

The Narconon websites (drugrehab.org.au) for Australia and (drugrehabus.org) for USA, are full of helpful data and have links to more information and uplifting testimonials from graduates. As you search be prepared to see discouraging information, it is certainly out there. But by using what you now know, it will be clearly obvious what is true and what is just black PR.

11

Final Thoughts and Conclusion

Having completed a proper and active detox, the metaphoric angel has now returned, and this time she is standing strong on *both shoulders*! This is the first time, since the first drag of a joint, or sniff of a powder, that the angel is no longer in competition with the metaphoric devil that unfortunately always wins the battle when drugs are involved.

Now the drugs are completely removed, the metaphoric devil is also removed. The students can look at him, size him up, and understand that everything that he whispered was wrong, selfish, hurtful, and morally corrupt.

The students learn to be able to face the devils of their past and no longer feel any shame or guilt. They realize that they had been manipulated and their thinking twisted by the force of the addiction and that now with the drugs gone and with the new skills they have acquired they are truly free to live again.

Whether it was people that they thought were friends, peer pressure, depression, or just 'experimenting', the students will learn that they were essentially hustled and robbed of their better judgment. They were certainly given the wrong solution to whatever it was that was that was troubling them when they started using.

They learn that it was not a matter of right or wrong or a matter of morals. They learn it was the difference between making a survival choice or a non-survival choice. Destroying oneself with drugs is very non-survival to oneself. Cheating on others and stealing from them also weakens their survival.

Looked at from a survival point of view it is much easier to decide what to do in any given situation. You can ask yourself this question: "Does what I am about to do make my survival better and those around me survive better too?" If it doesn't, it is not a good choice.

So now, with their newly learned skills, the successful student who graduates from the Narconon program can walk into the city again without hesitation.

Armed with confidence and knowledge the following situation will no longer be a problem: Walking along, the student sees an old drug using (former) friend, who may offer a taste of the baited hook of temporary pleasure, "just for old time's sake..." The graduate now knows exactly what is going on and will be able to respectfully decline without the slightest temptation. After all, the graduate now knows this person is not a true friend, and he also knows with absolute certainty the offer will not bring lasting pleasure but enduring pain instead.

The graduate now has no need for what is being offered. They have resolved the reason they got into drugs in the first place. They are stronger and much wiser now. The once hidden toxins, now gone, are not able to unknowingly and unpredictably resurface. They are not able to influence the person because they have been flushed out during the active detox. Because of what they do in phase two the graduate is able to think clearly about the consequences of every decision they make.

Yes, by completing the two phases of the Narconon program – first the active detox, and then the life-changing learning process and enlightenment that follows – your loved one will no longer be a walking, talking relapse waiting to happen. They will have regained their self-respect and newfound confidence in themselves without any hang-ups from past shame or guilt. They have become true to themselves again.

They are not different people than they were before drug use, but rather a new, improved, stronger and more capable version of themselves. They will be someone even more powerful, because of what they have learned. They will have the opportunity to finally live a sober life and the infinite possibilities that are part of a healthy, sober life. Most importantly, they will have become the best, most able versions of themselves with a confidence they may have never achieved otherwise. They will go on to be able to form better friendships, have greater opportunities, and live an overall better life than they ever thought possible.

The fact is, it is possible, and not all that difficult. The only hard part of the Narconon program is actually getting involved (if you could say making a phone call was hard).

Since this book has been aimed at family members, friends, and spouses of addicts, deeply worried about their loved ones, I urge you to re-read any portion of the information I have presented and think hard about it. If you are looking for a way to help your loved ones overcome a very difficult time in their lives, it may not be that easy. There are many choices available to you. The thing is, none of them are really going to work in any long-term way unless they do the detox properly and take the person through an effective life changing phase.

The life changing phase must result in a complete change of attitude and the acquisition of skills for effective living. Without these life skills they can fall prey to old habits.

For over 40 years these techniques have been employed and have continued to amaze those who experience them - both the successful student and their friends and family alike. Before entering the never-ending circle of failing treatment models and relapses please consider what is at stake.

Don't listen to anyone who tries to tell you that there is no way out. Such discouragement is not only flat-out wrong, but it is another blow to the hopeful spirit who needs help. Take the knowledge and findings I have provided here and let them guide you on your mission to save the life of your loved one. Reach out for more information about a local Narconon program, talk to other graduates or staff and give your loved one the greatest gift that could ever exist: the chance to be completely released from the chains of addiction, and to return to a happy, healthy life with unlimited possibilities.

If you are deeply concerned about your loved one, you now have the real story, the facts that slip by too many desperate families, friends and spouses. Please take advantage of what I have related to you. The power is now yours, so take advantage of this newfound power of knowledge and realization. You *can* save your loved ones life, and it will be the best decision you ever made.

That is obviously why I wrote this book. You will find that, in addition to saving the life of *your* loved one, you can also help save the lives of many more people out in the world – who like you, were once lost and discouraged.

You have no reason to be discouraged any longer. Be hopeful and confident now that you know the whole story about treatment and what does work and what does not.

Far too many people are dizzily spinning in a circle of treatment and relapses – you *can* help to put an end to this circle of suffering and hopelessness.

You *can* help stop drug addiction from continuing to spread.

It has taken away the hopes, dreams, and even lives of far too many already. This deadly epidemic must be ended, and the Narconon program is the only one I have found that can end this unnecessary suffering - *once* and *for all.*

More at:

drugrehabus.org

drugrehab.org.au

youtube.com/archiesview

End

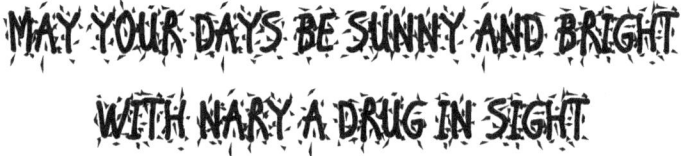

MAY YOUR DAYS BE SUNNY AND BRIGHT
WITH NARY A DRUG IN SIGHT

Disclosures and Disclaimers

When this Book is published through Amazon.com or Kindle reader devices and software neither the Author nor the Publisher makes any claim to the intellectual property rights of Amazon.com, its subsidiaries, or related entities.

All trademarks and service marks are the properties of their respective owners. All references to these properties are made solely for editorial purposes. Except for marks actually owned by the Author or the Publisher, no commercial claims are made to their use, and neither the Author nor the Publisher is affiliated with such marks in any way.

Unless otherwise expressly noted, none of the individuals or business entities mentioned herein has endorsed the contents of this eBook.

Limits of Liability & Disclaimers of Warranties

Because this book/eBook is a general educational information product, it is not a substitute for professional advice on the topics discussed in it.

The materials in this book are provided "as is" and without warranties of any kind either expressed or implied. The Author and the Publisher disclaim all warranties, express or implied, including, but not limited to, implied warranties of merchantability and fitness for a particular purpose. The Author and the Publisher do not warrant that defects will be corrected, or that any website or any server that makes this book available is free of viruses or other harmful components. The Author does not warrant or make any representations regarding the use or the results of the use of the materials in this book in terms of their correctness, accuracy, reliability, or otherwise. Applicable law may not allow the exclusion of implied warranties, so the above exclusion may not apply to you.

Under no circumstances, including, but not limited to, negligence, shall the Author or the Publisher be liable for any special or consequential damages that result from the use of, or the inability to use this book/eBook, even if the Author, the Publisher, or an authorized representative has been advised of the possibility of such damages. Applicable law may not allow the limitation or exclusion of liability or incidental or consequential damages, so the above limitation or exclusion may not apply to you. In no event shall the Author or Publisher total liability to you for all damages, losses, and causes of action (whether in contract, tort, including but not limited to, negligence or otherwise) exceed the amount paid by you, if any, for this book.

You agree to hold the Author and the Publisher of this book/eBook, principals, agents, affiliates, and employees harmless from any and all liability for all claims for damages due to injuries, including attorney fees and costs, incurred by you or caused to third parties by you, arising out of the products, services, and activities discussed in this book, excepting only claims for gross negligence or intentional tort.

You agree that any and all claims for gross negligence or intentional tort shall be settled solely by confidential binding arbitration per the American Arbitration Association's commercial arbitration rules. All arbitration must occur in the municipality where the Author's principal place of business is located. Arbitration fees and costs shall be split equally, and you are solely responsible for your own lawyer fees.

Facts and information are believed to be accurate at the time they were placed in this book/eBook. All data provided in this book/eBook is to be used for information purposes only. The information contained within is not intended to provide specific legal, financial, tax, physical or mental health advice, or any other advice whatsoever, for any individual or company and should not be relied upon in that regard. The services described are only offered in jurisdictions where they may be legally offered. Information provided is not all-inclusive, and is limited to information that is made available and such information should not be relied upon as all-inclusive or accurate.

For more information about this policy, please contact the Author at the e-mail address listed in the Copyright Notice at the front of this book.

IF YOU DO NOT AGREE WITH THESE TERMS AND EXPRESS CONDITIONS, DO NOT READ THIS BOOK.YOUR USE OF THIS BOOK, PRODUCTS, SERVICES, AND ANY PARTICIPATION IN ACTIVITIES MENTIONED IN THIS BOOK, MEAN THAT YOU ARE AGREEING TO BE LEGALLY BOUND BY THESE TERMS.

Affiliate Compensation & Material Connections Disclosure

This book may contain hyperlinks to websites and information created and maintained by other individuals and organizations. The Author and the Publisher do not control or guarantee the accuracy, completeness, relevance, or timeliness of any information or privacy policies posted on these linked websites.

You should assume that all references to products and services in this book/eBook are made because material connections exist between the Author or Publisher and the providers of the mentioned products and services ("Provider"). You should also assume that all hyperlinks within this book are affiliate links for (a) the Author, (b) the Publisher, or (c) someone else who is an affiliate for the mentioned products and services (individually and collectively, the "Affiliate").

The Affiliate recommends products and services in this book/eBook based in part on a good faith belief that the purchase of such products or services will help readers in general.

The Affiliate has this good faith belief because (a) the Affiliate has tried the product or service mentioned prior to recommending it or (b) the Affiliate has researched the reputation of the Provider and has made the decision to recommend the Provider's products or services based on the Provider's history of providing these or other products or services.

The representations made by the Affiliate about products and services reflect the Affiliate's honest opinion based upon the facts known to the Affiliate at the time this book/eBook was published.

Because there is a material connection between the Affiliate and Providers of products or services mentioned in this book/eBook, you should always assume that the Affiliate may be biased because of the Affiliate's relationship with a Provider and/or because the Affiliate has received or will receive something of value from a Provider.

Perform your own due diligence before purchasing a product or service mentioned in this book.

The type of compensation received by the Affiliate may vary. In some instances, the Affiliate may receive complimentary products (such as a review copy),

104

services, or money from a Provider prior to mentioning the Provider's products or services in this book/eBook.

In addition, the Affiliate may receive a monetary commission or non-monetary compensation when you take action by clicking on a hyperlink in this book/eBook. This includes, but is not limited to, when you purchase a product or service from a Provider after clicking on an affiliate link in this eBook.

Health Disclaimers

As an express condition to reading to this book/eBook, you understand and agree to the following terms.

This book/eBook is a general educational health-related information product. This book/eBook does not contain medical advice.

The book/eBook's content is not a substitute for direct, personal, professional medical care and diagnosis. None of the exercises or treatments (including products and services) mentioned in this eBook should be performed or otherwise used without clearance from your physician or health care provider.

There may be risks associated with participating in activities or using products and services mentioned in this eBook for people in poor health or with pre-existing physical or mental health conditions.

Because these risks exist, you will not use such products or participate in such activities if you are in poor health or have a pre-existing mental or physical condition. If you choose to participate in these risks, you do so of your own free will and accord, knowingly and voluntarily assuming all risks associated with such activities.

Purchase Price

Although the Publisher believes the price is fair for the value that you receive, you understand and agree that the purchase price for this eBook has been arbitrarily set by the Publisher. This price bears no relationship to objective standards.

Due Diligence

You are advised to do your own due diligence when it comes to making any decisions. Use caution and seek the advice of qualified professionals before acting upon the contents of this book/eBook or any other information. You shall not consider any examples, documents, or other content in this book/eBook or otherwise provided by the Author or Publisher to be the equivalent of professional advice.

The Author and the Publisher assume no responsibility for any losses or damages resulting from your use of any link, information, or opportunity contained in this book/eBook or within any other information disclosed by the Author or the Publisher in any form whatsoever.

You should always conduct your own investigation (perform due diligence) before buying products or services from anyone offline or via the internet. this includes products and services sold via hyperlinks embedded in this book.

105